MW00331211

BECOMING YOU

Create and Live an
Extraordinary Life

Mona Shibel

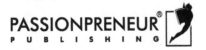
PASSIONPRENEUR®
P U B L I S H I N G

Publishing information
Publishing, design, and production facilitated by Passionpreneur Publishing, A division of Passionpreneur Organization Pty Ltd, ABN: 48640637529

www.PassionpreneurPublishing.com
Melbourne, VIC | Australia

Contents

Testimonials

Mona is an amazing coach and mentor who inspires by example. She is full of wisdom and always follows her own guidance. Her ability to manifest her best life is truly inspiring. She doesn't only share concepts, she helps you see what is possible for yourself by watching her own manifestations. I highly recommend Mona if you would like big shifts in your life – she is truly inspirational!

— Alison, Canada

What year better than 2020 to know that you can get help with getting through it? That's what Mona offered me, as it was a year that not only brought COVID-19 but heartbreak for me. I owe it to Mona, who showed me how to vibrate onto what I want to live and not what I call "reality," and I'll never forget the words "reality is what we create." Thank you, Mona.

— Nuhad, Lebanon

Mona is a powerful manifester who has created lots of great results for herself in her life, and this has really inspired me to do the same. I have really benefited from her services, and I love to watch the universe unfold.

— Francesca, UK

Mona has helped me manifest money and feel good about paying my bills! First, I was having super-high bills, especially after my daughter was born, and she provided me with guidance on how to shift my mindset each time I paid a bill and it really stuck with me, and within no time, I was paying my bills with great ease and no stress. Even though they were much higher (10 to 20 times as much as they had been) as my income grew, I felt completely at ease. Then there was another time when my husband was driving and we were talking on the phone and he was discussing this 91k that was due that day for some business payment and cash flow was behind for some reason. And I told him to manifest, just like Mona told me, and, seriously, within 30 minutes, exactly 91k was paid to us by someone that we weren't expecting!

— Erica, US

To Mom and Dad

Thank you for your unconditional love and for always supporting my passions and decisions.

CHAPTER 1

Becoming Me

From Breakdown to Breakthrough

—◆▦◉ ◉▦◆—

In 2002, when I was in my late 20s, I suffered a severe anxiety attack.

I was living in Beirut, Lebanon, at that moment in my life, and there was nothing wrong in particular that warranted panic, but at the same time, in the core of my being, I was incredibly unhappy and didn't know why. While I had a lot to be grateful for and I had my family and friends around me, as well as health and a good job at a reputable bank, it was far from what I intuitively knew was the life I was meant to be living.

The most difficult aspect of it was not knowing who I was meant to be and what else I could be doing. I did not actually have a reference point. All I knew was that I was not myself. Wherever I looked, I felt uninspired by what I saw. I knew what I did not want, and it was all around me. I tried to use my mind to come up with something new, but this led to a complete dead-end.

I was judged by my work colleagues for being too weak. In hindsight, I now know that everything in our reality reflects our inner beliefs, and I was actually judging myself.

I asked myself: *What right do I have to suffer? There are people who can't put food on their table. There are people experiencing true loss and tragedy. There are people who have lost their health and would be blessed to have my life.*

What I eventually learned is that any form of suffering should not be discounted. And this dismissal of pain is the precise reason that people end up suffering even more. They believe that they are not entitled to be unhappy when they have a good life compared to others. Yet, every person has a unique journey, and one should always compare apples to apples; that is, where you are versus where you would prefer to be. It's never about comparing oneself to others.

Suffering does not only involve experiences of tragedy and physical sickness. I was suffering a loss of spirit for choosing a life that was not mine. This is more common than not and shows up in people through various physical and mental ailments, including anxiety and depression, chronic pain, and, at times, more severe and deadly diseases.

According to the World Health Organization, 300 million people around the world had depression as of 2017. That's 4% of the world population.

> *"People suffer when they pursue a life … that doesn't belong to them."*
>
> — Caroline Myss, *Anatomy of the Spirit*

What I didn't know was that this low moment in my life was a blessing in disguise. It was my inner spirit demanding a change.

In that state of panic, my mind finally surrendered and pleaded for help. In that moment of surrender, I allowed for something bigger and more powerful to take charge of my path. My physical mind was no longer behind the wheel.

Within the weeks and months following that incident, life shifted for me in ways I could not explain. Everything that I experienced from that point forward was leading me to a path of becoming more myself. The people I met, the experiences I had and the knowledge I learned all played vital roles.

I took some time off from work. The transformation started slowly. In moments when I was feeling better, inspiration would come to me. This was new, as I had not been inspired for years. I would get random calls from interesting companies for job interviews. This would give me a glimpse of another career possibility. Later, I was approached to do freelance consulting work for a media company, which was a line of work that was completely fresh and different, and I was able to apply my unique skills to help that company. New people started coming into my life that helped lift me up energetically. They were positive and inspiring. They showed me what was possible.

It was like a doorway opened slightly and I could peek into the field of possibilities.

Then one day, at the bank where I worked, all employees who worked in credit were required to attend a one-month intensive training course in finance. But this training was to be delivered gradually over a period of 1.5 years. My colleague attended the first batch of training, and I was due to attend the second batch in September.

My direct supervisor, with whom I'd always had a great relationship, didn't think I should attend this batch because my colleague was on leave and there was a shortage of staff. It was an understandable reason so I didn't resist.

To my surprise, my boss at a higher level suggested I attend the training despite the shortage of staff. It was so out of character and unexpected of her to make that suggestion. I did not get along with her and she always triggered me in ways that no one else had in my career up to that point.

With time, I came to realize that the people who trigger you the most, whether in a positive or negative way, are always your soulmates. You make spiritual contracts with them to help direct you and keep you on your intended path. As odd as it may have sounded to me at the time, I now know that my boss was definitely a soulmate.

I went ahead and attended the training, which was divinely orchestrated for me in several ways.

During that training, something in me shifted dramatically. For the first time, as I observed the trainer and his approach, I felt that I could be good at training others. In fact, it was evident to me earlier than that, but I never really paid attention. Whenever we had interns join our bank, I was happy to teach them and guide them. This training opened up the "door of possibilities" wider. I felt extremely inspired and excited. But I rested in that feeling without taking any action.

One day, a few weeks later, I received some new inspiration from my brother in Dubai. He spoke of the success and recognition he received less than one year into his new job through a promotion and financial bonus. As this was not the first time I'd heard of such success stories from people living in Dubai, it inspired me to consider moving.

Interestingly enough, both my brother and sister lived in the UAE. So did one of my long-time best friends! Yet, this was the first time I felt inspired to move. It felt good to consider this move. It didn't feel "heavy" or out of reach, as it may have felt in the past. As I considered this option, it shifted from just an idea into an actual decision.

I remember telling my best friend about my decision to move to Dubai, even though there was still no job prospect nor anything feasible to hold on to. I remember her saying – having been in Dubai for many years – that it may take some time to find employment. But for some reason, I felt this would not be the case.

I had a confidence that I could not explain. I somehow felt "supported" in my decision. I had unwavering belief that I would get a job. I did not know how, but I knew it from the depth of my being.

Then, suddenly, I got an exciting idea. I decided to email the owner of the Dubai-based training company that had run the training at my bank two months earlier. I reached out to him hoping he might know of any companies hiring. He worked with many banks and, surely, would have some contacts. Having excelled at that training (because I was inspired and unknowingly in high vibration!), he actually remembered me. To my surprise, he offered to hire me himself. Just like that.

> *Your higher mind always has a bigger,*
> *grander vision.*

Two months later, I moved to Dubai.

Looking back, I now know that my move to Dubai was divinely orchestrated and divinely supported. In my moments of hesitation as to whether or not I should move (our fear-based ego mind craves security and comfort), three people pushed me forward: my brother, cousin, and best friend. Both my cousin and best friend were very close to me, and I spent a great deal of time with them living in Beirut, yet they both unselfishly pushed me to move forward.

My move changed my whole life's trajectory and it's the reason why I am where I am today. The job I got gave me so many opportunities to learn, grow and excel. It was a complete shift in energy to an environment where anything and everything was possible. My boss, who remains a friend to this day, treated me like a partner, not an employee. Everything I experienced in that job was what I was unknowingly craving.

At times, my ego mind would get activated and want to assert itself through negative thoughts, emotions and patterns, as the ego thrives on pain. Yet, intuitively, I learned to shut it up and say, "No, no, there's no place for you here."

The more I learned to shed and disidentify with my ego, the more of me started to shine through, and people noticed.

Riwa, a good friend of mine from Lebanon, was amazed at how different I seemed. I recall her saying, on one of my visits back to Beirut, that I seemed like a new person. At the time, I didn't have an answer as to why I was different. But now I know that I had learned to disengage with the inner chatter of my mind. And my overall vibration was much higher.

About two years after moving to Dubai, my good friend Erica told me about a book called *The Secret*. She said there was a new fascinating book that claimed you can have anything that you want. I was so intrigued; I went out and got it the same day and read it cover to cover in one go.

At an intuitive level, the concept fully resonated with me. I knew it to be true. I recalled the circumstances around every time I got something and every time I didn't. *I knew* it was *true*.

While the book was a great starting point, I knew there was much more to it. In a matter of weeks, I went on to read many more books on the topic and started to remember and laugh at all those times in my past when I had unknowingly manifested things and thought it was coincidence. Of course, we are always manifesting and it's not something we need to learn. But I did notice the cause and effect in various scenarios in my life up to that point. In fact, my move to Dubai was an example of a perfect manifestation although I did not know it at the time.

In one of the books I read, the author proposed testing the Law of Attraction. The exercise said that I must set the intention to receive something that, when it happens, I will know that it cannot be coincidence.

I will never forget the day I set the intention to receive an email from a high-school friend. We kept in touch but very sporadically. We'd reach out to each other every few years. I didn't even remember the last time we connected. So receiving an email from her at this time could not be coincidence. I first thought about manifesting an email from her on a Sunday and then forgot about it. By Tuesday, I had recalled the intention and refocused on it. I had email notifications enabled on my laptop and imagined her email popping up on the bottom right-hand side of my screen. I focused on it, imagined it, and then closed my laptop and went to sleep.

The next morning, I opened my laptop and, lo and behold, the email notification from my friend popped up on the bottom right-hand side of my screen, exactly as I had imagined it would the night before. The timestamp on the email was 12:02 am, just three minutes after I had closed my laptop the night before. I was in shock. I couldn't stop laughing. I could not believe it. She said that she saw my sister on Facebook and was wondering if I had a profile on Facebook. It was just when Facebook was becoming popular, and I didn't even have an account yet. Needless to say, the universe put my sister in front of her so that she would be inspired to reach out to me.

This first conscious Law-of-Attraction success story makes me smile to this day.

My eagerness to learn more about how manifestation works gradually started to expand my understanding and consciousness to a deeper spiritual level. I was ready for the second part of my journey, and a new scene was going to be the place for it.

Again, I now know that it was divinely orchestrated. A few years ear-lier, when I was still living in Beirut and right before I moved to Dubai, as I "followed my joy," I took some salsa lessons as part of following my excitement.

When I moved to Dubai, I dropped it for about two years. In that time, I would get the idea on a recurring basis to get back into salsa dancing. But I didn't take action on that idea.

Then one day, towards the end of 2006, I coincidently met an old-time friend at a party. He happened to be the DJ hired for that party. Out of the blue, and quite randomly, he told me about a weekly salsa night that I should attend. I heard it – as I had gotten the idea a few times – but still didn't "get around to it."

Then a few weeks later, my best friend was told about the same salsa night but from a completely different person, who was a work col-league. Hearing this twice, over and above my own idea to start danc-ing again, I took action with my two best friends.

Looking back, I have no doubt in my mind that this was divinely orchestrated through the inspiration, and then, consequently, through two different people.

Sometimes, you will be inspired to do something.
If you don't take action, you will hear the call
from different people.

Going to salsa was certainly a fun experience, and it is a hobby that I enjoy to this day. But it was more than that. Over the next 10 years,

I would meet several people that have unknowingly played an instrumental role in my spiritual development. Through my interactions, I was able to let go of old beliefs that were no longer serving me so that I could start afresh and imprint new, more empowering beliefs. I also encountered people who triggered me immensely. I started to identify the work of the negative ego and how it operates. Some experiences relating to those people inspired desires within me that would not have been born otherwise. I reached a whole new level of understanding of spirituality, manifestations, and the nature of physical reality, all of which I will be sharing in this book. Essentially, that salsa scene paved the way for me to write this book.

> *Every desire you have and every action*
> *taken in joy is leading you on the path of*
> *becoming more yourself.*

Simultaneously, through the years, I learned to follow my joy in every moment. And in doing so, my path unfolded before me every step of the way. I was inspired to start a business in 2008, in a field completely different from finance. I took that inspired step not knowing that it would lead me to where I am today.

The business I started also had nothing to do with what I am doing today but it was my stepping stone for what was coming next. I learned more about what I preferred and what I didn't prefer. With every new step, I learned more about myself, allowing something new and exciting to unfold.

I can list for you all the wonderful manifestations and creations I experienced but would not necessarily be able to inspire you with them because I learned that everyone is here to express themselves in their own unique way. What inspires me and brings me to life may not be the same for you. The particulars of my life, which invigorate me, may not invigorate you.

The key is to live a life that excites YOU, and only you.

What I can tell you is that during my shift in awareness as I came to understand that we are the creators of our own realities, I took several big, bold steps in my life. Steps I would not have dreamed of just two short years earlier. I started two different companies. I quit my full-time job. I manifested fabulous clients, fun and interesting work colleagues, new, like-minded, spiritual friends (my manifestation buddies) and exciting and meaningful projects.

I have been self-employed since 2011, living without the constraints of a full-time job. My days are mine to plan. I have manifested a life that is exactly what I personally desire.

This book, in this moment, is my true joy. I am not writing this book because I consider myself an authority. I am writing it because as I've learned to disidentify with my mind and to become more my true self, I feel an inner tug to express all this in some form. This is part of my excitement. It's my truth and my passion in this moment.

But the problem is that most people have a very restricted definition of success. I once hired a marketing expert to help me sell an online coaching program. I shared with him all the amazing (to me!) experiences that I had manifested and were thrilling to me. He dropped everything (literally) and only used the external factors that he thought people wanted to see. Basically, he only focused on the money and the freedom.

This is not to say he was wrong, as that is what moves people. The problem is that, in doing this, we are living by society's definition of "success."

It's the reason why so many people are so unfulfilled and experiencing chronic pains and ailments. We live in a society that is massively concerned with external factors, such as wealth, lifestyle, and material things, putting an undeniable strain on people to pursue careers that fill their bank accounts but deplete their souls.

It's time to redefine what true success means.

Don't get me wrong. Financial abundance is also wonderful, and you will attract it very naturally as a by-product of being authentically yourself. But it shouldn't itself be the end goal, not because money is evil, and you should not want it. On the contrary! Financial abundance is your birthright. But in focusing on money as an end in itself, you might be compromising on your passion, as the physical mind has a limited perspective on how the two can be mixed.

It is understandable that people still want to know that they will be supported if they follow their dreams and become more authentically themselves. The fear-based mind needs the reassurance. The answer to this question is a definite yes. You absolutely will be supported. I've lived this since 2011. If you surrender control from your physical to your higher mind and if you let go of subconscious limiting beliefs – both of which we'll be covering in this book – you will absolutely be supported financially.

But to live a truly fulfilling life, you must not let the abundance be the driving factor. Let your inner fulfillment and passion be your end goal, and the abundance will naturally come.

Recently, I watched a TV interview in which French DJ, record producer and songwriter David Guetta shared how he followed his passion never knowing nor imagining that he would one day achieve the massive success that he has. He was just following his joy, DJing at parties and mixing music. By doing that, he eventually sold over 50 million records globally and his music has had 10 billion streams. If financial abundance was his driver, he would never have started. Until David Guetta paved the way for others to do the same, it had been unheard of for a DJ to achieve this level of success. His end goal was not the sales. His end goal was just to work with music because that was authentically how he wished to express himself. It was his passion and joy.

As I share later in the book, you have to learn to disidentify with the fear-based ego, whose instinctive job is to keep you safe. If you allow your higher mind to guide you, you will be led on the path of least resistance, which may not start with all the abundance you desire, but it will get you there (sometimes sooner than you think), and by then, it will not really matter because you will be so exhilarated on the inside as you express your passions that the outer abundance will just be the icing on the cake.

This is the true meaning of financial freedom. It is freedom from the need for financial abundance because true abundance is an abundance of passion, experiences, adventure, synchronicities, joy, connections, and fulfillment.

I hope by now you know that you are reading this book for a reason. Your soul brought this to you for a purpose because there are no accidents.

I just ask that you keep an open mind and allow your true self to emerge and shine, for that is what you were created to do and how you can choose to express yourself.

This life is your movie. It is your creation. You are the writer, lead actor, producer, and director of this movie. You decide what the script is. It is a blank slate for you to create yourself and your life in the best possible version.

Chapter 2

You Attract What You Are

No Ifs, Buts or Whys

→══◎ ◎══←

Are you falling short of living a truly authentic life? Have you attempted to live that life but have failed? Do you wonder if there is even another extraordinary life that you could be living? Have you experienced a multitude of achievements but still sense a void?

If you've answered YES to any of these questions, then the biggest and most important question I'd like to ask you right now is this:

Would you like to know how to become more YOU?

The first time my life changed forever was in 2006 when I learned about the Law of Attraction. The second time my life changed forever was a few short years ago when I learned that we each have our own signature vibration, which automatically attracts the people, situations and circumstances that will allow us to become more ourselves and live a truly extraordinary life. This vibrational quality is how, pre-birth, we chose to express ourselves in this physical reality. But we are preventing these manifestations from becoming visible in our reality by holding on to limiting beliefs and definitions.

In this book, I will be sharing foundational principles on who you really are and how you manifest your physical experience, followed by a formula for living a truly extraordinary life. This formula is so magnificent because there is no homework or extra effort required. You don't have to meditate for hours, unless you want to! You don't need to force anything or set goals or exert effort. You don't even need to set intentions, for your heartfelt intentions will always inherently revolve around being more yourself and you can achieve that just by following your joy.

The only thing you need to do is follow your excitement in every moment. Just by doing that, your spirit will take you where you need to go to live the extraordinary life that is your birthright.

The Missing Link

At the end of 2017, two of my friends were staying with me for a few days before leaving Dubai for good. As Law of Attraction fanatics, we were constantly speaking about manifestations and especially about Abraham-Hicks. As business owners, and me being self-employed, we had all manifested our desires enormously. But that year was a tough one financially and, while we avoided dwelling on it – as that would aggravate things further – it did, at times, elude us as to why there was still any struggle. Abraham-Hicks says, "If this time-space reality has the wherewithal to inspire a desire within you, it has the wherewithal to bring it about in full manifested form."

So having consciously LIVED this for over a decade, we all should have gotten the hang of it by then.

"I am not sure that the Law of Attraction actually works" were the words that my friend finally blurted out.

I didn't agree. How could I? We had lived it and breathed it for years. But I did hear what she said and started to wonder if perhaps there was a missing link.

I have read books by great teachers including Wayne Dyer, Louise Hay, Jerry and Esther Hicks, Deepak Chopra, Eckhart Tolle, Neale Donald Walsch, Gabby Bernstein, and the works of multiple individual teachers from *The Secret* including Bob Proctor, Jack Canfield, John Assaraf, Joe Vitale, Bob Doyle, Mike Dooley, Bill Harris and Michael Beckwith. I have also read some of the work of historical authors such as Napoleon Hill and Wallace Wattles. I've also listened to celebrities such as Oprah and Jim Carrey talk about how they've consciously manifested their lives. They all said – more or less – the same thing.

All of them have had an influence on my way of thinking when it comes to the Law of Attraction. Admittedly, the greatest influence has been the teachings of Jerry and Esther Hicks (Abraham-Hicks) and I must have listened to hundreds of hours of their teachings. I literally thought I knew it all when it comes to this topic, for the message was crystal clear – until I dug even deeper and came across various additional teachings. The most prominent of these were the teachings of Darryl Anka (Bashar) and Neville Goddard. Needless to say, truth is truth. The overall message is the same, but there were additional very important messages that really struck a chord with me and had me thinking.

They seemed to be "the missing link." Or at least, this was the first time I heard the message communicated in this way. These messages are tied to the following concepts:

1. Who we really are.

    Any time a spiritual teacher spoke about who we truly are, it was understood to mean that we are creators and spiritual beings having a physical experience. This is 100% true. However, there is a key element that seems to be missing in many of the teachings, and that is who we REALLY are. In this book, I will share what I have learned that to mean.

2. You manifest what you are.

    Many of the Law of Attraction teachers focus on teaching how to attract what you want, as if it is externalized. Contrary to that concept is "you attract what you are" and this has been a key message within the teachings of Wayne Dyer, Bashar and Neville Goddard.

3. Positive thoughts and positive vibration are not enough to manifest your desires.

    No matter how positive our thoughts may be and how high our vibration is, we may still manifest non-preferred circumstances that may seem the opposite of what we desire. Do not get discouraged because this is part of the manifestation process! There is a perfectly reasonable explanation for this.

4. Co-creation does not mean that we are creating together. It is always just me creating alone.

This is one of the biggest hang-ups in Law of Attraction that causes people to doubt that they can create anything they desire when there are other people involved. They question how they can "influence" others or cause others to change. If there's anything you can learn from this book, let it be this. You are always creating alone.

5. The term "Law of Attraction" is not an accurate depiction of how manifestation occurs.
   The use of the term "Law of Attraction" implies that we are attracting something outside of us or bringing something external into our reality. This is a flawed premise. The more accurate correct term is "manifestation," as I'll explain later in the book.

6. "Don't take action unless it's inspired" is extremely misunderstood.
   People think that aligned action is supposed to get you to your manifestation. It's 100% true but it may not be a direct path. The outcomes "in the middle" are just as important and have a higher purpose as well.

Learning this new information took my manifesting abilities to the next level. I am someone who likes to understand something conceptually to live it. I understood it previously, but I didn't always get the actual physical dynamics of how it worked. I worked on faith and then knowingness. But when you learn how it actually works, it will make perfect sense and take you to a whole new level of manifesting, becoming more of your authentic self and living the extraordinary life that is your birthright.

We are experiencing this physical reality to remember that we are creators, to experience the process of creation, and to align with our unique signature frequency and express that uniqueness. The process of unfolding all of that is meant to be joyful, exciting, imaginative, passionate, adventurous, curious, and extraordinary. It's not about a destination but about the journey of becoming more YOU.

There's no struggle required. In fact, your inner being will navigate you through your core beliefs and values using the path of least resistance. You won't suddenly be required to DECLARE something about yourself that makes you feel uncomfortable or uneasy. It is truly a gradual process that takes you, one step at a time, onto a path that unfolds before you and allows YOU to discover more about yourself. The process is truly invigorating because as you peel back the layers, you will feel more and more joyful in every moment, and everything will feel like an easy, natural next step.

We are living in a time when more and more people are living their joy. More people than ever are pursuing their passions and achieving great success in the process in the most traditionally unexpected fields, from multimillion-dollar raw food coaches to beauty experts growing their social media by the millions to international DJs achieving massive success mixing and creating music.

This is not to mention the miraculous stories of people creating health and recovery all around the globe, including Anita Moorjani, who fully and quickly recovered from advanced stage-4 lymphoma following a near-death experience to the complete surprise of her doctors. There are multiple stories of people recovering from chronic pains and diseases through healing meditations and breathing. Dr. Joe Dispenza has multiple such testimonials on his website.

The realm of possibilities has reached new heights and will continue to do so as the consciousness and awareness of our creative abilities continue to grow. Every one of us has the ability and capacity to create a more authentic life doing what we truly love.

We just have to say YES and allow our inner beings to guide us through this. Your feeling of excitement and passion is the indication that there is more of you wanting to express itself.

This book will take you, step by step, through an understanding of all these concepts and how you can effortlessly start to live a truly extraordinary life being more YOU.

The book is divided into three parts. The first part covers the foundational and core principles relating to who we really are (really!), how physical reality is structured, and how our physical mind works relative to our higher mind. These foundational principles will clarify how manifestation really works and how to follow the cues of the higher mind in order to manifest an extraordinary life.

The second part covers, step by step, how to start creating a life that is much more aligned with your authentic self.

The third and final part will cover how to deal with the non-preferred outcomes and circumstances that show up and how they are all part of your manifestation! So do not fret.

Part 1 – Foundational Principles
Chapter 3 – Who We Are

In this chapter, we will lay the foundation of who we truly are. What does it mean when we say: "Who we are"? It helps to start by identifying who we are not.

We will also go further into explaining who we are from a deeper spiritual level.

By understanding that we each have a signature essence waiting to be expressed uniquely through a new perspective, and how important a role you play in the expansion of the universe, you will start to understand how vital it is for you to live your life authentically as the YOU that you are intended to be.

Everything and everyone you experience and interact with in your life is coming to you based on your unique frequency, as you are automatically attracting to yourself all that is in resonance with who you are. You sometimes struggle to let these people, experiences, and situations into your life because of your negative beliefs and definitions.

On the flipside, everything in your life that is not in resonance with who you really are is there because you are holding on to it. Why do you do that? Again, because of your negative beliefs and definitions.

This is life-changing! It certainly was for me.

We'll also talk about your practiced vibration and how to better align with your true essence by raising your vibration and what tools and techniques would be helpful for easier alignment.

Chapter 4 – How Physical Reality Works

In this chapter, we will cover the meaning of physical reality, which is the physical world we experience in all its physicality. Is it really real? Or is it just a dream or illusion? We will focus on what it is, why we are here, and how physical reality actually and literally manifests through our subconscious minds.

It will also cover how we create the illusion of time and continuation and what happens when we "tune into" a higher vibrational frequency.

It is magical because you will learn that change is instant, and in every moment, you become a new you. The past never matters, and it doesn't matter who you were, for the present moment not only impacts the future, it also impacts the past.

Finally, we'll be talking about co-creation. Who are the people we are interacting with in our reality? It's a given that they are soulmates, but this chapter provides an even bigger understanding of what co-creation really means. We are co-creating, but the only vantage point that truly matters is YOURS and only your free will matters.

Chapter 5 – The Physical Versus the Higher Mind

In this chapter, we will talk about the physical mind and how it's different from the higher mind. Our physical conscious mind is very limited in perspective and has functions that allow it to perceive what has HAPPENED and not necessarily what will happen. By disidentifying with the fear-based physical mind – and its limiting thoughts – you allow the higher mind, which has a much higher and wider vantage point, to take the lead and navigate you through the path of least resistance.

We'll talk about how the higher mind communicates to you in physical terms. You don't need to go into meditation to hear it or feel it. It's always there guiding you, and only you disconnect yourself from it by allowing your physical mind to take control of the wheel.

The higher mind wants you to succeed because it's YOU. Your success is its success. It knows what your heart truly desires and it's holding your hand in every step to get you to your desires.

Finally, we'll cover the power of the conscious versus the subconscious mind, which is the whole basis for our physical reality, contrary to people's understanding that the conscious mind is in control. It isn't.

Part 2 – The Steps
Chapter 6 – Intend and Imprint

In this chapter, we will talk about how to set intentions the right way, so they imprint in the subconscious mind and, consequently, reflect outwards into our physical experience. Every intention set the right way is literally a seed being planted that must manifest.

We'll cover how this step of deliberately setting intentions raises our vibration and gets us excited about what's possible. However, whatever manifests will always be grander and better than what our physical mind could ever imagine.

Finally, we'll cover what to do after setting intentions as well as the role of the physical mind from there onwards.

Chapter 7 – Stay Present and Follow Your Joy

This is where the magic truly begins. This chapter brings a whole new meaning to inspired action. By following your joy, it becomes all about the journey. We are here to experience the process of creation, with its time lag. Going through the steps of following your excitement in every moment is what the creation process is about.

This also helps you stay present, enjoy the journey towards your manifestation – because every step of the way is a manifestation – and raises your vibration. Following your joy also gets your mind off the presence (or absence) of your manifestation. It's never about waiting for anything. It's literally the journey that is thrilling and exciting.

We'll also talk about how to disengage the physical mind in the process because it really doesn't know what the purpose of any aligned action is and where the higher mind is leading us. It will always be bigger and better than what's imagined by the physical mind.

Chapter 8 – Ride the Wave

In this chapter, we will cover the multiple elements of excitement, support and synchronicities that will be unlocked if you follow the steps of the previous chapter. You will learn about how to remain fully present and let go as the wave of excitement, synchronicities and support take over your life.

You will notice a surge of energy flowing through you so every action seems effortless and you'll be excited to wake up in the morning.

You'll learn about the elements of excitement and synchronicities and how to discern the difference between positive and negative synchronicities.

You will see how abundance will flow to you in divine timing and how to let go of how that will happen and in what form.

This is the most exhilarating phase because you will feel that something divine is being orchestrated in every moment. The key is to LET GO. Allow this phase to take you where you need to go. By trying to activate your physical mind, you will interrupt the flow. But it's not a problem because negative synchronicities will show you when a path is not yours. The key is to pay attention!

Part 3 – Dealing With the Outcomes
Chapter 9 – Circumstances Versus State of Being

This chapter covers the one thing that often takes people out of alignment and makes them discouraged about manifesting their desires. The circumstances that you manifest will sometimes appear as a non-preferred outcome – despite being in a positive space – but, in fact, every outcome is 100% leading you to your desire in its highest form. And, no, this does not mean getting something different from what you envisioned. It is getting what you want in its highest form, as will be explained in that chapter. The negative circumstances are only a step towards helping you align yourself to your own highest vibration by releasing beliefs that have no place in your preferred reality.

The key is to remain positive no matter what. Your current outer reality is truly irrelevant. Focus inwards and practice a positive state so that you can be clear on why a certain circumstance has manifested. Sometimes, it may even just be an echo of your previously practiced state of being.

Chapter 10 – Your Reflection

In this chapter, we will cover what beliefs are, how we come to adopt them, and how to release negative beliefs and reinforce positive ones. We'll talk about how belief systems work and how negative beliefs often work on reinforcing themselves. We'll also cover how to use powerful techniques for reprogramming your subconscious mind, which is the one and only aspect of us that manifests outward. No exceptions.

By working on these belief systems, your outer reality miraculously changes to match. The key is to remain humble in not knowing what beliefs you actually might be holding on to, regardless of how far you've come along on your journey.

PART 1

Foundational Principles

CHAPTER 3

Who We Are

Our Unique Essence and Perspective

⋅⇥▭◉ ◉▭⇤⋅

"Trying to be someone you're not is the most difficult
thing you can do in life."

— Bashar

To live a truly fulfilling life, we must let go of the burdens of who we perceive ourselves and others to be. To live in authenticity and be free to creatively express ourselves fully in the way our soul intended, we must shed the fear-based thoughts and beliefs that are the products of our instinct-driven ego mind. To live an extraordinary life, we must know "who we are not" in order to realize who we are and how inherently unique every one of us truly is. When we realize the extent to which our very existence enhances the whole of creation, we will learn that being fully and authentically ourselves is the best service we can provide for ourselves and others.

In this chapter, we will cover who we think we are versus who we really are. We'll cover how to become aware of our ego mind at work and how it's been designed to function; in this understanding, we can learn to disidentify with it. We'll also cover how we each have a unique signature frequency and each one of us is an important and crucial piece of "all that is" (i.e. the universe), which requires our unique perspective to be complete. Finally, we'll cover how we can align with our unique frequency and say YES to becoming more of our true selves.

⋯▸▬◉ ◉▬◂⋯

Who We Think We Are

When asked who we think we are, most people tend to have a similar yet limited perspective. They refer to what they do for a living, their qualifications (it helps when they have a qualification that comes with a certain title), their talents, and a list of other self-perceived characteristics that they believe enhance their identity. And if going deep, and opening up, they speak of the traumas and experiences that may have "defined them," adding to that the deep beliefs that they have about themselves that don't feel good.

Essentially, who we tend to think we are is an egoic mask composed of all the external factors that we choose to give meaning to and identify with, meshed with deep-rooted inner beliefs we have about ourselves and how we think people perceive us.

Our illusory sense of identity is usually composed of (a) an internal self-image, which represents everything we believe to be true about ourselves, including our intellect, physical and personality traits, and inherent and learned talents; and (b) external self-image, which comprises external considerations we choose to identify with, including our possessions, achievements and reputation.

> *"In normal everyday usage, 'I' embodies that primordial error, a misperception of who you are, an illusory sense of identity. This is the ego."*

> — Eckhart Tolle, *A New Earth: Awakening to Your Life's Purpose*

As part of the internal self-image people have of themselves, they tend to strongly identify with their minds and all the thoughts and beliefs that are persistently, repetitively and, at times, uncontrollably active within them. They do not separate themselves from these thoughts and all their accompanying emotions.

The Ego Mind

To understand who we are, we must first understand the ego mind in order to learn to disidentify with it.

> *"The path of awakening is not about becoming who you are. Rather it is about unbecoming who you are not."*

> — Albert Schweitzer

Our ego mind is where all the thoughts and beliefs about who we think we are stem from. It is fully conditioned by the past.

As described by Eckhart Tolle in his book *A New Earth: Awakening to Your Life's Purpose*, the ego mind consists of content and structure.

Content represents all the things we have learned to identify with based on conditioning from our environment, upbringing, and surrounding culture. This could be where we're from, who our family is, our schools and universities, educational level, our achievements, career, assets and an endless list of things we choose to identify with.

Structure represents the ego mind's innate need to identify with an object, believing that it will enhance its identity. In fact, the very basis of the ego's existence is "identification," and it is very much needed in the physical experience in order to separate "me" from "not me" (having come from oneness, as I'll explain later).

This structure is the same for every individual. What changes is the content and what people identify with.

Most people are highly identified with the content of the ego mind, which is fear-based because its very existence is required for survival of the "I" and, therefore, much of the inner chatter of the ego mind – the thoughts and related emotions – is often focused on a comparison of "my content" to "other people's content," and will frequently remain in a self-critical state.

Disidentifying with the Ego Mind

To disidentify with the ego mind, one must become aware of the thoughts and emotions as they are happening. In doing so, and holding still long enough in this observation, you can become conscious of an inner presence within you (which is your soul or spirit) that is separate from these thoughts and emotions.

> *"Spiritual realization is to see clearly that what I perceive, experience, think, or feel is ultimately not who I am..."*

— Eckhart Tolle, *A New Earth*

At times, when you are still for long enough, you can hear the loving voice of your spirit (i.e. your higher mind).

> *"The spirit is the part of you that feels like hope."*

— Caroline Myss, *Anatomy of the Spirit*

With practice, you can start to discern the voice of the ego from the voice of the spirit, which has a multitude of ways to communicate with you including through the physical sensation of excitement and passion, as we'll cover in Chapter 7.

The qualities of the ego mind and the spirit can be summarized in some of the following ways:

Ego Mind	Soul/Spirit
Critical and judgmental	Loving and compassionate
Fear-based	Has faith
Compares itself to others	Focused on one's individual and unique journey

Ego Mind	Soul/Spirit
Driven by pride	Driven by love and joy
Concerned with self-image (Reputation)	Concerned with self-expression, uniqueness and authenticity
Regretful	Always present in the now and forward-looking (past is irrelevant)
Victim-oriented	Self-empowered

With time, it will become easier to release our attachment to the illusory egoic mask, inclusive of both the internal and external self-image we have become so identified with, because of our awareness of the indestructible and loving spirit within us. Plainly, it just feels better to separate ourselves from our egos.

This is when we provide ourselves with the opportunity to release the burdens and confines imposed by the ego mind of what is required and expected of us in any given moment. This is when we can start to live a free and expansive life full of endless possibilities.

Who We Are

Awareness of that inner presence within us is a great starting point to identifying with who we really are.

The unique expression of who you are is for you to discover through your individual life's journey, for the very purpose of life is to discover who you were created to be based on your unique signature frequency and to express yourself in that way.

But at a fundamental level, we are all infinite spiritual beings having a physical experience. We all come from one consciousness (creation, source energy, "all that is," the universe, etc.) and we are all creators of our physical reality.

From this one consciousness, we split into individuated souls, each with a unique signature frequency or energy stream. We came into this physical experience with no memory of our origin and who we were created to be, with the intent of remembering who we are and experiencing that through a new perspective. It is a path of pure self-discovery, and if life is lived out in that way – and if we see ourselves as that spirit and not that critical ego mind – it can be a truly thrilling and fulfilling experience.

This is not a spiritual quest. It is very much a physical quest because we are spiritual beings having a physical experience, not the other way around. We came into this physical reality to explore, expand and evolve, for it is through these perspectives that creation's awareness of itself also expands.

Think of the non-physical "spiritual realm," which is where we all come from, as the realm of understanding yourself from a theoretical perspective (the school), while the physical realm, which is where we are currently focused, is an understanding of yourself from an experiential perspective (the job), and is where true expansion, growth and discovery can happen.

Your Unique Signature Frequency

Although we all come from the same place, and we all have the same creative powers, each one of us is unique and came into this physical experience to express ourselves differently.

Each person has his/her own unique vibrational essence (or frequency). Think of it as the soul's DNA. It is an energetic quality that is unique to you.

This signature vibration does not change. However, your expression of this frequency can change, and it's unique to you because your expression of it is different from everyone else's. It's your unique reflection as an expression of creation.

As you go through the process of discovering yourself, you will find different ways of expressing that signature frequency, and to do so more fully, you must let go of the fear-based beliefs that cloud your ability to accomplish this.

Creation needs you to be fully you because every individual is like a puzzle piece with its own unique shape, which fits perfectly into the big picture puzzle of creation. By trying to be a shape that you're not, you do not help in the creation of the big picture.

You Attract What You Are

Through the Law of Attraction, like attracts like. Therefore, you automatically and unconsciously manifest the people, situations and experiences that match your unique vibration (provided your beliefs and definitions are not getting in the way). Because these people, situations and experiences are aligned to your unique frequency, they will flow to you very naturally and you will feel completely in sync, happy, and fulfilled with those inter-actions and experiences. There is nothing that you actually need to practice or do. You are automatically doing it through your unique vibration.

As Bashar puts it, you are like a lighthouse beacon automatically attracting things to it and the only reason that experiences that are aligned with your vibrational essence are not showing up is because you are holding them away with your beliefs and definitions. And any experiences that continue to show up for you that are not in alignment with you are there because you are not letting them go. This is also because of your beliefs and definitions.

Generally, you will see some evidence of your unique qualities through-out your life. If your unique qualities include an engagement with public speaking, then you would have seen evidence of that earlier in your life. For example, as a student, you may have done well in school presenta-tions, or you were part of the debate club, or people were always drawn to your conversations. If you have immense fear of public speaking, it may also be an indication that it's part of your unique vibration because if it's not in your vibration (and it wouldn't be for someone if it's not rel-evant to them), you wouldn't even think about it, unless you have chosen a path that is not yours.

It's not just one quality such as singing or painting. And it is certainly not just an artistic trait. It's a mesh of various natural inner qualities that are unique to you, and come very naturally to you. In fact, often, they come so naturally, you do not realize that they are a gift and you think everyone else can do them the way that you do.

You may also be drawn to seemingly unrelated things. One client of mine was drawn to multiple unrelated activities involving talent acquisition, beauty makeovers and aviation. It caused her some confusion because she couldn't see how they were all linked and a representation of WHO SHE IS. But there is always a bigger picture that we may not perceive with our physical mind. These are all clues to your unique vibrational frequency, and in Chapter 7, we will cover how you can follow your joy in every moment and allow your life to easily unfold so you can express all your gifts naturally.

The important point is to not compartmentalize or categorize, as we typically do. We live in a world where we are taught to nurture a limited number of gifts or talents; otherwise, we are considered scattered and "lacking in focus." But that is a limiting perspective. It's never about this OR that. It's this AND that. It's a mesh of various inner qualities that are here to be expressed. That's what makes YOU incredibly unique.

By following the formula of Chapter 7, the path will unfold before you in a way that allows you to uncover these unique qualities and what's completely relevant to you. Do not try to figure this out using your physical mind. It will be highly limiting to do it in this way for reasons I'll explain in Chapter 5.

No Comparisons Are Ever Required

Many years ago, Oprah spoke on TV about her experience when she first started the *Oprah Show*. At the time, Phil Donahue was a massive success and was named the "king of television."

She stated that, when she was recruited to start her own morning TV show in Chicago, where Donahue's show was also being broadcast, the management of her station told her not to worry about Donahue because they knew it would be "impossible" for her to beat him. As a result, she stated that she never felt any pressure to be like Donahue and was encouraged to just "be herself."

That was probably the best advice one could give to someone because just by being herself, within just a few months, Oprah's show had 100,000 more viewers than Donahue's and was the first in terms of ratings.[1]

Being uniquely YOU means never having to be like anyone else.

As Bashar puts it, being uniquely YOU means not comparing yourself to others because this would not be comparing apples to apples.

> *"You are a very particular perspective of the infinite and there is absolutely no other point of view like yours. Your uniqueness should never be invalidated or devalued by comparing yourself to someone else."*
>
> — Bashar

Creation requires your uniqueness in order to be "all that is." The unique properties that are YOU are required in order for creation to

---

1   Oprah Winfrey – Quotes, Facts & Network – Biography

experience all that it can be. Otherwise, it would not be complete and infinite.

Our individual frequencies make up the WHOLE, and every soul contributes to the fullness of "all that is."

In conclusion, you are not your ego mind. You are an infinite spiritual being having a physical experience, and you are here to express your signature essence from your unique perspective. By becoming more of yourself, you will perfectly fit into the big picture puzzle of "all that is" (creation).

Your State of Being or Practiced Vibration

Your signature frequency is extremely high. In order to align with it more fully, it would be helpful to work on uplifting yourself, although the steps covered in the book will automatically help you raise your vibration.

Your state of being or practiced vibration is a reflection of your general vibrational attitude and how you're feeling in any given moment.

You can know what your practiced vibration is by how you mostly feel at an emotional level. Are you mostly in an emotional state of worry and doubt or contentment and hopefulness?

The emotional vibrational scale is composed of 22 energetic frequencies tied to the various human emotions, as shown in the table below.

THE EMOTIONAL VIBRATIONAL SCALE

1	Joy/Knowledge/Empowerment/Freedom/Love/Appreciation
2	Passion
3	Enthusiasm/Eagerness/Happiness
4	Positive Expectation/Belief
5	Optimism
6	Hopefulness
7	Contentment
8	Boredom
9	Pessimism
10	Frustration/Irritation/Impatience
11	Overwhelm
12	Disappointment
13	Doubt
14	Worry
15	Blame
16	Discouragement
17	Anger
18	Revenge
19	Hatred/Rage
20	Jealousy
21	Insecurity/Guilt/Unworthiness
22	Fear/Grief/Depression/Despair/Powerlessness

Source: Adapted from the book *Ask and It is Given* by Esther Hicks and Jerry Hicks

As you go up the emotional scale, your state of being or practiced vibration increases, getting you closer to your unique signature frequency. As a result, you feel more connected to your inner being.

The lower down you move on the emotional scale, the more you feel a sense of "separation," although you are never separated from your inner being. You just feel like you are. In that state, you are essentially in a practiced state of resistance; you are in misalignment and resisting your natural unique vibration. Simply put, you don't feel good, although it's important not to confuse sensitized emotions for "normal."

As you move up the emotional scale, you automatically attract to you the things that match your signature frequency whether you are conscious of it or not. On the flipside, as you move down the emotional scale, you can't see the "light." You doubt yourself. You wonder if you are good at anything. You're out of ideas. You're simply disconnected, and you're more likely to make more fear-based decisions. This is exactly where I was when I experienced my anxiety attack.

As you feel more of the positive emotions, you are more in alignment with WHO YOU ARE, and you will keep going up the emotional scale as you go with the flow and allow the universe to bring you the people, experiences and situations that are aligned with your core vibration.

When you are consistently high on the emotional scale, you will find it difficult to choose a path that is chosen by the ego. You will just not resonate with it. You will feel the misalignment immediately. In your high vibration, your true path becomes so much clearer. You will feel the resonance of who you are authentically.

In your low vibration, you follow the cues of the fear-based ego because you are in fear and you, therefore, activate your survival instincts.

This would not be the time to create! Or you may feel doubt and start requesting external validation from other people, although you always have your own guidance within you. When your vibration rises, you will tend not to seek any other person's validation or approval. You know and trust your inner guidance.

Think about how you typically feel in any given day. This may require conscious awareness because it may be such a practiced feeling that it almost feels natural or "normal." Think about it. What emotion is it? Is it anger? Is it frustration? Is it blame? Or is it well-being, contentment, and optimism? If you practice moving up the emotional scale and remaining in those good-feeling emotions (without reacting to the environment), you will make a habit out of it. It will become natural for you to be like that. You will find it difficult to feel any other way.

I remember when I changed my diet a few years ago and stopped eating sugar and flour (I literally read the label on everything), any time I cheated after that, I would get a horrible headache. This is what it will feel like for you once you clean up your vibration. You will find any negative emotion to be horrible and, at times, intolerable.

You are naturally in a state of well-being. Think about how you feel when you first wake up, and before you start activating your thoughts. You feel good. But you keep choosing to bring yourself down by thinking about what you don't want and/or reacting to your environment.

> *"Every choice you make either enhances your spirit or drains your spirit."*
>
> — Caroline Myss

In Chapter 7, we will cover an extremely easy process for you to raise your vibration in a natural way. It is so easy and so powerful, but it will require practice and persistence to not be in a reactive place. You cannot keep reacting to your environment if you want to reach your true potential.

Becoming More You

By understanding conceptually who you really are, you push the door wide open to realigning with that vibrationally and expressing yourself authentically.

In doing so, you will always manifest what you need or what's relevant to you at any given moment in time.

What's relevant to you will be what will help you get closer to your core vibrational frequency. This means that you will attract people, experiences or situations that will help you (a) raise your practiced vibration; (b) raise your awareness to limiting thoughts, beliefs and patterns that you may be holding on to; and/or (c) release attachments that may be blocking you from moving forward.

At times, it may feel like you're moving further away from what you want, but, ultimately, the seemingly longer route will help you get what you want in its highest form faster.

Essentially, by letting go of ego mind control, the universe will automatically help you to become MORE YOU. And you will attract the people, experiences and situations that will joyfully help you on that journey.

Your purpose in life is to become more and more aligned with that unique vibration. The remainder of this book will be focused on a further understanding of how our physical experience works to get us closer to our true vibrational essence and how we can go about easily navigating through our limiting inner thoughts and beliefs to fully express ourselves in the way our soul intended.

I would like to end this chapter with an excerpt from the book *Dying to Be Me,* written by Anita Moorjani, who experienced a near-death experience (NDE) and came to the realization – in the spiritual realm – that she still had a purpose to fulfill in her life. Although she had the choice to return or not, she chose to return to her body to fulfill her mission. Here's what she had to say about her realizations during her NDE:

"If feels as though I have a purpose of some sort yet to fulfill …
I perceived that I wouldn't have to go out and search for what I was supposed to do – it would unfold before me. It involved helping lots of people – thousands, maybe tens of thousands, perhaps to share a message with them. But I wouldn't have to pursue anything or work at figuring out how I was going to achieve that. I simply had to allow it to unfold.

To access this stage of allowing, the only thing I had to do was *be myself!* I realized that all those years, all I ever had to do was be myself, without judgment or feeling that I was flawed. At the same time, I understood that at the core, our essence is made of pure love. *We are pure love* – every single one of us. How can we not be, if we come from the Whole and return to it?

CHAPTER 4

How Physical Reality Works

Everything Is Me, Projected Outwards

⊷⊨⊙ ⊙⊨⊶

"Everything is energy and that's all there is to it. Match the frequency of the reality you want and you cannot help but get that reality. It can be no other way. This is not philosophy. This is physics."

— Albert Einstein

If a tree falls in a forest, and no one is around to hear it, does it make a sound? You have probably heard this philosophical question before, and it may have gotten you thinking.

Yet, this is not just a philosophical question for it is also an observation raised by quantum physicists. Why is this relevant to you?

Read on to find out why.

This chapter will help you understand how manifestation is working in every moment. When you understand the nature of reality, you will get how you are truly the creator of everything you see in your physical world. We will be covering how, according to quantum physics, physical reality does not exist separately from the observer (you). It is an illusion and a projection of your state of being and inner beliefs. Change yourself and you must change the projection.

We will also be covering how everything already exists because we live in an infinite universe. Every thought, idea, situation, and circumstance already exists. You just tune into those things by changing your practiced vibration. Through your experience of these thoughts, ideas, situations, and circumstances, you are expanding creation's awareness of itself.

The chapter also covers how everything is now and our concept of linear time is an illusion. Every moment is a frame or snapshot and is a projection of our vibrational state of being. Every moment, we shift to a new parallel reality based on that new state of being. This means that no matter where you have been, you have the opportunity to create a new, more preferable reality for yourself in any given moment. The past does not matter and only exists in your own memory.

You're not the only one shifting through parallel realities in every given moment. The earth, the universe and the multiverse are also shifting. By focusing on a vision of a preferable earth (whatever that may be for you), you are tuning into a reality where that must be the case.

You'll also learn about the nature of desires, for any time a desire is born within you, you are tapping into a physical reality in which a version of you is living that desire.

Understanding Is Key

For all these years since I came to understand how manifestation works, I have had a good understanding of key concepts around manifestation. But some of the information I share with you in this chapter, in particular, I did not know until recent years. This was the main reason I felt drawn to write this book because it was a huge A-HA. Now that I truly get it, I know that the world is my oyster. Everything is truly possible because this life we are living is our movie and we are the lead actor, writer, director and producer. Every single person we interact with is a supporting actor, and a bunch of "extras" are also there to provide the random people we see in our world. All of them are waiting for our cue on how to script the plot and play out the movie.

In the book *The Secret*, there was an emphasis on how it's not really important to understand how the Law of Attraction works, in the same way we may not understand how electricity works.

Yet, electricity is proven. If I switch on the light switch, the light comes on. I don't need to understand how and why that works in order to light up my room.

However, when it comes to bringing the invisible into the visible, an understanding of how this all works helps in opening our minds to the immense possibilities. Knowing the basics of manifestation is greatly empowering but believing and, ultimately, knowing (through our own experiences) how far we can stretch our reality is where true expansion and massive shifts take place.

Physical Reality Is an Illusion

According to quantum mechanics, the observer is critical to physical reality. This means that without an observer, reality does not exist. It is an illusion and is only created by the consciousness of an observer.

So not only does a tree not make a noise in a forest when there is no one there to hear it fall, the whole tree and forest do not exist if there is no one present to perceive them.

This is what is truly meant by the concept of physical reality being a projection of you. It is a projection of your inner world. It is your reflection in the mirror and would not exist if you were not there looking at it.

You came into this physical experience to create and remember who you are. The physical reality that you interpret with your five senses is projected outward in such a way to make it seem as real as possible. But it really is just make-believe.

It is only a movie in which you are the star actor, writer, director and producer. The movie script is written by you, whether consciously or subconsciously. When you are aware that you are the creator of your reality, you are writing the script consciously. When you are not aware, then you are writing it unconsciously, based fully on your past experiences and inner beliefs.

But what actually plays out — whether you wrote the script consciously or unconsciously — is impacted by both your state of being (your mood at the time the movie is being created) as well as your inner subconscious beliefs.

This means that it's not enough to consciously script the movie but — as the lead actor, director and producer — you must also remain in a positive state as the actual movie is being created. When you are angry and frustrated, the actors will also mirror that back to you through their actions and behaviors. They will be disgruntled. They will be difficult to please. They will be impossible to deal with.

If you're mostly in a positive state, but your actors keep going off-script and behaving in a way that is not to your preference, or things keep going wrong on the set, then that is a clue to you that you may have subconscious beliefs within you that are creating those scenarios. The key is not to get angry at the actors but to remain in a positive place and dig within yourself to uncover what those beliefs are so you can clear them and start manifesting the desired behavior from the actors.

Through this analogy, you can understand how reality is a projection of your state of being and subconscious beliefs in any moment. In this book, your state of being is defined as how you're feeling emotionally in a moment of time (refer back to the emotional scale in Chapter 3). It's your vibrational attitude. Change your state of being first and then you will see the changes in your physical reality. It can't be the other way around.

Your subconscious beliefs also play an important role. If — despite your positive state of being — you are manifesting non-preferred circumstances, then you must go within to see where changes need to be made. We will be covering this more deeply in Chapter 10. For now, start to consider what negative subconscious beliefs may be responsible for the parts of your outer reality that you do not prefer.

Co-creation

This is your universe. Any person you are interacting with in your universe is your perceived version of that person. You are not interacting with their souls directly, but only a version of them that you have created – by agreement – in order to interact with them. And they are doing the same with you in their universe, which is a completely parallel version of reality that is unrelated to the reality you are creating here and now.

So, essentially, all the people you are interacting with are your supporting actors (your parents, siblings, spouses, friends, boyfriends/girlfriends, bosses, colleagues, clients, acquaintances, etc.). From your perspective, in your movie, they are all waiting for cues and instructions from you on how your movie plays out.

Every person that you are interacting with is mirroring back to you where you are vibrationally (your practiced vibration) and what subconscious beliefs are present. They reflect back to you those inner beliefs and definitions.

If you are unhappy with the actions and behaviors of another person, perhaps with your spouse, your boss, or your mother, consider what subconscious beliefs within YOU are creating the other person's behavior. No one is ever doing anything to you. You are the only person responsible for every action or behavior you see from others. When you truly get this, you will never blame another person for anything ever again because you will know that you are 100% responsible for the creation of that behavior from others. It is incredibly empowering.

Anything You Focus on, You Activate

If there are people, situations or circumstances that you do not want to include in your experience, then shift your focus away from them. Do not give them any attention or focus whatsoever.

Oftentimes, we place a great deal of energy and focus on the issues we do not prefer. However, by doing that, we are activating them in our reality. Literally. We are causing them to remain visible in our reality. Remember, physical reality does not exist separately from the observer.

Think of it in terms of your movie. Would you create sets for scenes that you have chosen to delete from your script? Would you hire actors to play roles in those deleted scenes? So then why are you hiring those actors and building those sets by giving them attention? This is essentially what you are doing when you focus on unwanted things.

However, if you have truly shifted your focus away from them, and with time, they continue to show up, then there must be some inner beliefs causing them to manifest. This is where you would dig deep into what may be the cause of that manifestation.

It is also important to understand that many of these situations are also present in our experience for the sake of contrast, as we'll cover at the end of this chapter. You cannot know what you want unless you are also clear on what you do not want.

Everything Already Exists

Everything already exists. Every thought, idea, and invention. You are never creating anything new. They are just currently "invisible" to you. These only become visible when you tune into their frequency, as physical reality does not exist separately from the observer.

You tune into that frequency by changing your vibration, which can be achieved by following your joy.

Although everything already exists, your experience of that reality is what's new and that's how creation expands its awareness of self.

How is this relevant to you? It is relevant in letting you know that any time a new desire is born within you, that desired reality already exists. Everything you want exists. You just need to tune your perspective into that reality. You do not have to create anything or attract anything outside of you. By shifting your perspective, you shift your reality.

Everything is Now

Not only is your physical reality an illusion, but the concept of linear time is also an illusion, since everything is happening now. Your past, present and future are all happening at the same time because everything in reality already exists. What is changing, and giving the illusion of linear time, is your perspective of that reality.

How is this relevant to you in manifesting? Since everything is now, the past does not matter. It does not matter where you have been.

What remains active of the past is only your memory of it. By understanding this key point, you will realize that it does not matter what has happened in the past, what you did or did not do, and what you perceived were past traumas or misfortunes. Everything is happening now, and every moment, you have the opportunity to create a new physical reality based on your current state of being.

In the next section, we will cover the concept of parallel realities, and this further reinforces how your past is completely irrelevant because you literally become a different person in every moment.

Parallel Realities

Even though we perceive movement in our physical experience (similar to a movie), every millisecond, we are shifting into a new parallel reality. Think of it as a "snapshot" or frame in an old-fashioned movie.

Every millisecond, you are experiencing a new snapshot. It's happening so fast that there is the illusion of continuity. In the same way a traditional movie is created through a series of frames, so is your reality. Every frame is a snapshot of a given moment and is reflective of your state of being in that moment.

This means that every moment, you are a new person. You are shifting through billions of parallel reality versions of yourself and the earth every second. You don't need to learn how to shift as that is happening automatically through the concept of time, space and change. You just need to become aware of the fact that you are always shifting and start to match the frequency of the shift more closely. As you do this, you become more present in the moment.

The earth, universe, multiverse and creation are shifting as well. This shifting extends throughout existence. You, as an individual, are shifting on a planet that is also shifting because it is one of the parallel versions that you have shifted to.

When you practice remaining in a positive emotional state (through your practiced state of being), you will start to see the effects of these shifts in your physical reality even while you are still witnessing the old reality. As you do this, for some time, you may see evidence of both the old and the new realities. This is truly miraculous because while you see the shift into a more preferred reality, you may still see signs of the old one happening simultaneously.

This is when you become conscious of the shifts happening, and you may see an overlap between multiple realities through a "residual echo" of the reality you are shifting from and another "residual echo" of the reality you are moving to. This is especially the case where the earth is itself shifting because, for some time, you may still see the turmoil happening in certain parts of the world while seeing great progress and well-being in other parts.

Through this overlap, as Bashar explains it, you are seeing the non-preferred reality through a "glass wall." You may see it, but it will not impact you unless you choose to invite it into your reality.

This is how true manifestation works, for you are not attracting something outside of you to you. You are tuning into a parallel reality that is more reflective of your vibrational frequency.

The key is to observe the undesired reality without reacting to it. This is the big tipping point that allows you to fully cross over to the new reality without wobbling back and forth or re-inviting the old reality back into your experience. It's similar to crossing a bridge where you can see your previous reality and you can also see the upcoming reality from the same bridge. The important point is to keep moving forward on the bridge towards your desired reality by remaining in a positive space.

When you react negatively to the non-preferred reality, you are walking back on the bridge towards the non-preferred reality. Literally!

You Are a Different Person

Do you ever look back at old photos and find it hard to grasp that you are the same person? This tends to be more a positive interpretation (although for some, it may not be), for you have grown and changed so much that you find it difficult to identify with the old you. This is not just perception. This is real. You are not the same person, not physically nor spiritually nor from a literal parallel-reality perspective.

Physically, you are a completely new person, for the vast majority of the cells in your body fully replace themselves periodically, so that within a few months, all cells have replaced themselves. The exceptions are the lenses in your eyes and most neurons of your central nervous system. You are literally a different person.

From a parallel-reality perspective, as you shift to a new preferred version of yourself in a parallel reality, the past corresponding to that version must also change. To have created that preferred present and future version of yourself, you cannot also be the same person of the past. Your present not only creates your future, it also changes the past, for that past version of yourself was vibrating at a different frequency and had a very different life trajectory.

For example, had I not had that anxiety attack and surrendered, I would not have ultimately shifted my vibration and manifested a new life in a new country. I would still be living that life at the bank. This is what is referred to as a timeline. I would still be in a timeline where I am living that life.

This means that by changing yourself now, both your past and your future selves also must change. The only one who is holding on to the undesired past version of yourself is you.

Unless you choose to make your undesired past relevant and invite it back into your experience, the past is completely irrelevant and holds no value whatsoever for where you choose to go. Your present and future possibilities are unlimited.

Every change is a total change and nothing that has happened to that other person (you of the past) can define who you are today. Every moment is a fresh slate.

Nature of Desires

Any time a desire is inspired within us, we are close to a parallel reality where a version of us is living that desire fully. There are infinite parallel realities and universes and, as mentioned earlier, everything already exists. Every thought, idea, invention, song, story, life experience and scenario already exists in a parallel reality. When a desire is born within us, we are vibrationally close to a parallel version of ourselves where that desire is fully manifest, and we are living it in full. How amazing is that?

Let this provide you with the confidence that anything you desire is absolutely possible. Otherwise, you would not have perceived that desire to begin with.

> *"If this time-space reality has the wherewithal to inspire a desire within you, it has the wherewithal to bring it about in its full manifested form."*

> — Abraham-Hicks

As you go through life, your experiences will inspire new desires and preferences. It never stops and it never ends. That is the purpose of our physical experience; our purpose is to expand and grow, and we do this by peeling back more and more layers of ourselves, and through that, launch even more desires. In this way, our awareness is continuously expanding and allowing creation's awareness of itself to expand through us.

Contrast Is Required for Expansion

Contrast is the observation or experience of something unwanted in order to determine what is wanted or preferred. Any time we are viewing something unwanted (such as war), we are automatically desiring the opposite (i.e. peace). Our desires are born out of life experience and are not always inspired by positive experiences.

That is why there is this polarity or duality in our physical experience. In order to expand our awareness of the light, we may need to experience the dark. War exists so that we can perceive peace. Sickness exists so we can know and appreciate the meaning of health. Poverty exists so we can appreciate abundance. Diseases exist so we can find the cures. And the list goes on.

It is important to understand that sometimes, even when you are in a positive space, you may attract something that may appear unwanted, and this is a part of the expansion of your awareness of what you do prefer and want. That is how you can learn more about yourself and what direction you prefer to take in life.

Let that be a natural part of your growth and do not get discouraged because it is all part of the unfolding of your path. By knowing what you do not prefer, you can gain greater clarity on what you do prefer so you can then divert yourself in the direction of higher preference.

→▬◎ ◎▬←

In the next chapter, we will talk about the differences between the higher and physical minds and how to hand over the reins to our higher mind. In doing so, it takes us on the path of most joy and least resistance on our journey of becoming more ourselves and manifesting our dreams and desires.

CHAPTER 5

The Physical Versus the Higher Mind

Mind, Be Quiet

—◦▨ ▨◦—

"Your soul knows the shortest, safest route to your true destiny. Why is your ego behind the wheel?"

— Anthon St. Maarten

In this chapter, we will cover the differences between the higher and physical minds. Our conscious physical mind is a perceiver of what has already happened in our reality, while our higher mind is a conceiver of it. Our higher mind, given its vantage point, can see the big picture. Being focused on the non-physical, it has access to multiple dimensions of reality, and uses that to guide us to a more preferred reality using the path of least resistance. The problem is that most people are relying on their physical mind – which has a very narrow perspective based on what it has experienced in the past – to navigate through physical reality.

We will also cover how our higher mind communicates with us through the physical sensation of excitement and is always guiding us in every moment. Our higher mind knows us better than we know ourselves, for it has been tracking our preferences through every single experience we have ever had. It is using this to guide us to the highest form of any manifestation.

We will learn the difference in the manifesting power of our subconscious mind versus our conscious mind. Contrary to what many people think, the conscious mind is not in control, for everything that manifests is a full projection of our subconscious mind.

Finally, we will cover how everything is energy and what the energetic layers of the human energy field are, starting from the lowest, most dense to the highest, most powerful which is representative of our soul's frequency. This will be useful to better understand vibration and how you can raise your own vibration for stronger and more consistent access to your higher mind.

When I started my first business, back in 2008, I was following my long-felt passion of starting my own business. I took that first step, not ever imagining that it would get me to where I am today. I followed my excitement, and each step of the way, the path lit up before me. In my first year of establishing my business, I worked with a business coach on the team of John Assaraf, who is one of the teachers featured in the book *The Secret*. This opened my eyes to the world of coaching, and I felt immensely drawn to that. I knew in my heart that, one day, I would be helping others consciously manifest their realities, and that my business was my learning ground.

Six years later, I felt it was time to move on to coaching, as my existing business was no longer an expression of my truth. But I had contracts that were binding me to an investor who had invested money into my business, so I couldn't just walk away. I remained in a positive space and felt excitement over my newly established business, which I moved forward in creating.

I shared my desire to step away from my existing business with a close friend, Alison, who fully understood my decision as she was also part of my journey and saw the direction that my life had been taking. She asked me what my plan was and how I was going to get out of this. As she probed, I felt a sense of unease and my body contracted because I really did not have the answer, but I knew that it would somehow work itself out. I told her that I did not have a plan and I was going to allow this to unfold.

About 10 days later, I was invited to a meeting with the investor. The representative shared with me that the market was moving into very tough terrain and they needed to withdraw from our arrangement. As he shared with me the reasons why they needed to break the contract, feeling like he needed to convince me somehow, I was in complete amazement. We amicably ended the partnership, one that was bound by obligations and legal clauses. Just like that, I was free to move on to my next chapter.

When I shared this with Alison, she laughed out loud and said, "How is that possible?!!!"

It would have been hard and quite impossible for me to conjure up a plan had I relied on my physical (logical) mind. Even when my friend had been asking me, I felt myself contract because I could not see how that was possible. So I "let it be," knowing that a path would open up somehow because the reassuring voice of my higher mind told me to trust that it would.

And it did. There was zero effort in the way it happened. It just came to me so effortlessly. I did not try to make it happen. I did not force anything. I did not plan anything. It came to me.

The Physical Mind Versus the Higher Mind

Throughout this chapter, I will be using the terms "ego mind" and "physical mind" interchangeably. This ego mind represents our logical, rational, thinking, analytical mind. It is also our conscious mind. It's the same ego mind we use for identification.

Bashar describes the physical mind as our "physical persona, which is made up of our beliefs, emotions and thoughts that create the ego structure and exhibit our behavior in physical reality."

As mentioned in an earlier chapter, we all come from one consciousness ("source energy" or "all that is") and then split into individuated souls, which have their unique signature frequencies or energy streams and come forth to experience a new perspective in physical reality. The ego mind is the structure that focuses the soul in a way that allows it to experience physical reality through three-dimensional space and one-dimensional time.

Bashar uses the analogy of a diving mask to describe the ego mind. If you dive into the ocean, it is going to be quite blurry unless you wear a diving mask that sharpens the image for you. That is the role of the ego, which allows you to see under water (i.e experience physical reality), but you do not rely on it for navigation or to direct you to where you need to go next.

That is not its job.

The physical mind's only job is to PERCEIVE. It has analytical and reasoning capabilities in relation to what has happened in the past but not for what can happen in the future. On the other hand, the higher mind's job is to CONCEIVE.

The higher mind, which is often referred to as our inner being, spirit, soul, or higher self, is the part of us that remains focused on the non-physical as a representation of the spirit vibration. It is the individuated soul that has split itself from the whole in order to create a physical reality experience but it remains in the non-physical.

The physical mind experiences a unique and distinct physical reality defined by three-dimensional space and one dimension of time. It only perceives what it has experienced in this time-space reality. The higher mind, which also has its own realm, has a fuller experience of multidimensional time (multiple realities, past, present and future) while the sense of physical space is not required for its experience.

This means that the higher mind can navigate in multi-dimensions of time through various parallel realities. It experiences past, present and future all at once since all realities are happening now. This point of view provides the higher mind with a broader big-picture view that allows it to guide the physical mind through its three-dimensional space and bring about the manifestation through inspired action.

Essentially, the higher mind has access to the quantum field or field of infinite possibilities.

The definition of the quantum field, according to Dr. Joe Dispenza, "is an invisible field of energy and information—or you could say a field of intelligence or consciousness—that exists beyond space and time. Nothing physical or material exists there. It's beyond anything you can perceive with your senses."

Every individual who has ever created anything – from music to art to the kind of "genius" work created by Mozart and Einstein – has tapped into this quantum field of infinite possibilities. This is always through the work of the higher mind.

Your higher mind knows your physical experience and perspective extremely well because it is YOU. It knows every detail about you: what fulfills you, what repels you, what makes you happy and joyful. And it has kept a record of all that on your behalf as you have experienced life, and based on your unique frequency, you will attract all the experiences that resonate with who you are at a core level, if you just let go of the physical mind's limitations. Your higher mind has the capacity to stretch you much further than your physical mind ever can.

What is considered the "best scenario" by the physical mind is actually the "worst scenario" of the higher mind. That is because the physical mind has a very limited perspective. It is bound by beliefs and definitions. It is externalized and tends to look outside itself for validation, acceptance, inspiration and ideas. Its perceptions are drawn from the past and, consequently, it can only create from the past. It has only one point of view, being any experiences perceived within its own physical reality.

"You cannot create anything new from the known."

— Dr. Joe Dispenza

By listening to your higher mind, which communicates to you vibrationally through the physical feeling of excitement and passion, you will be guided by a big picture vision. You will be able to express your true life purpose and manifest your desires as fully as you can. In doing so, you live a life that is extraordinary, ecstatic, expansive, joyful, curious, imaginative and loving.

Most people experience struggle because they try to plan out their life and manifestations using the physical mind. They try to figure out how to make things happen. The mind will often object and come up with reasons for why it can't be done. That is what I felt when my friend asked me how I planned to move away from my existing business. I felt the resistance of my physical mind.

If it is able to come up with a plan, the physical mind may try to explore a shorter route, but it may be much more difficult to navigate through, and it often will come up against multiple roadblocks. The ego mind, being fear-based, may also choose a known undesirable route over an unknown route because of its need for knowledge and control. The physical mind over-analyzes, tends to be in a needy state, and may try to manipulate and hold on fearfully to any opportunity. These are all effects of the negative ego.

People have been taught to burden the ego with the role of navigating through life, and as a result, start to experience the negative ego as a manifestation of a resentful ego that is doing a job it's not made to do.

The Conscious Mind Versus Subconscious Mind

People often think that the subconscious mind is lower than the conscious mind, thereby giving the latter a sense of control. However, it is the other way around. The unconscious and subconscious minds are both higher than the conscious mind in vibrational frequency and, consequently, our unconscious thoughts and beliefs have greater manifesting power.

In fact, anything that is imprinted into our subconscious and unconscious minds is reflected out into physical reality.

This means that even if you consciously believe that you can manifest something, and you are in a positive state, if it's not showing up in your reality, then there must be some unconscious beliefs related to the situation that are preventing the manifestation.

Likewise, if you imprint something into your subconscious mind using subliminal affirmations, or by visualizing or imagining with emotion (which we will be discussing in Chapter 6), you will manifest it, even if at a conscious level you do not believe it. I will repeat this point for emphasis. **Even if you do not believe it at a conscious level.** But the key is to not dwell on it consciously. You have to forget about it. Drop it.

How is this possible? Through techniques to imprint positive beliefs into your subconscious mind. I will show you these techniques in Chapter 10.

Essentially, it doesn't matter what the conscious mind thinks, whether positive or negative. The power is all, and purely, with the subconscious mind. The key is to not keep the limiting thought active within your conscious mind but to just forget about it.

Unlike the conscious mind, which has analytical and reasoning capabilities, the subconscious mind has no ability to analyze or determine whether something is possible or not. It's non-judgmental and non-selective. It is literally just the projector of what's inside it and what's given to it. It also does not differentiate between a real experience and imagination. It is only fed the experiences through thoughts and emotions. It does not know what is happening in the physical world. It is unlimited in its nature and its limitations only stem from what you feed it.

If a positive message is imprinted in the subconscious mind using the right techniques, the creation process begins through the workings of the subconscious with the higher mind, and in time, the manifestation has to become visible in your physical reality. No exceptions.

Your subconscious mind is responsible for your entire physical reality and everything you have experienced so far. Therefore, in the same way you have created everything in your life, both wanted and unwanted, you now have the capability to deliberately create your new life.

Our unconscious beliefs always generate thoughts, emotions and behaviors as well as reflections to reinforce the validity of these beliefs. In Chapter 6, we will be discussing how to imprint new positive images, and in Chapter 10, we will discuss how to release negative beliefs. These two steps, together, will ensure that the subconscious mind has what it needs to project out your desired reality.

Satisfying the Ego

As human beings, we often need to have a sense of where we are going and to feel that we have some control. This can be achieved by creating intentions, which represent the "what" or the "vision" of where you see yourself going. Essentially, it's what we will imprint into your subconscious mind in the next chapter. The "how" can then be dropped because it is not within the capacity of the physical mind to know how things will unfold or the quickest route of least resistance to follow.

If you are setting intentions from a pure heart space, then you are most likely tapped into your authentic self and your intentions will be a very close representation of experiences that will fulfill you. If, however, you are relying on the ego mind, and trying to intellectualize your intentions, then your manifestations may not necessarily fulfill you.

> This happened to me when I started my coaching business. In my gut, I wanted it all to be about spirituality and manifestation, but I intellectualized my decision and decided to rely on my ego mind when making the decision. I decided to do traditional business coaching because that was my background on all levels. I studied business, I worked in business analysis through my experience in credit and consulting, and I had started and run my own online business.
>
> So, of course, my logical "fear-based" mind chose the "known" path and I went into business coaching. It made so much sense that anyone I would have discussed this with would have agreed! But that was not what my heart was calling me to do. Choosing that route did not fulfill me in the way I had hoped it would. Yet, I have no regrets because now I know the difference between intentions set by the ego mind versus the higher mind, which will always direct you towards what will fulfill you and may not necessarily make logical sense in the moment.
>
> What your heart calls out to may not always make logical sense.

Raising Your Vibration

In this final section, I'll be covering some tips on how to raise your vibration. While it's important not to force anything, these are just some tips to help you remain mindful of what is impacting your vibration, as it is not just your thoughts and emotions.

Everything in the universe involves the movement of energy, some of which is high and fast while some is low and slow.

The material or physical world is the slowest moving energy. It's what we perceive as mass and form through our eyes and fingers.

Your physical body is part of this material world and its energic frequency can be measured. However, the physical body we see with the eyes is just one of the energetic layers that make up the human energy field. The remaining energetic layers, collectively called the person's aura, surround the physical body and may not be easily seen by the human eye. These energetic layers are where our physical, emotional, mental, and spiritual characteristics are stored. All of them impact our vibrational frequency.

1. Physical:
   As mentioned, the physical body's energic frequency can be measured and this is done using a BT3 frequency monitoring system that was invented by Bruce Tainio in 1991. The frequency of energy is measured in hertz, and frequency is the number of oscillations (movements) of an energy wave per second.

The average vibrational frequency of the healthy human body is within the range of 62-80 MHz, with someone in good health averaging 70 MHz. Studies show that human cells start to mutate when they drop below 62 MHz. When you have a cold or flu, your body frequency will drop to 58 MHz, while 42 MHz will be the frequency of the body when there is cancer. Death begins at 25 MHz.

There are several ways to help raise or maintain your physical body's vibrational frequency. Here are some examples:

Food. Food also has its own vibration and has an impact on the vibrational frequency of the human body.

Highly processed foods, which have a frequency of zero hertz, can actually lower the healthy body's frequency. Whereas unprocessed natural foods found in nature such as fresh food and herbs vibrate at 20-27 hertz, as shown in the food pyramid on the next page.

That is why you will feel sluggish when you eat processed food and much more refreshed and energetic when you eat healthy, wholesome, living food.

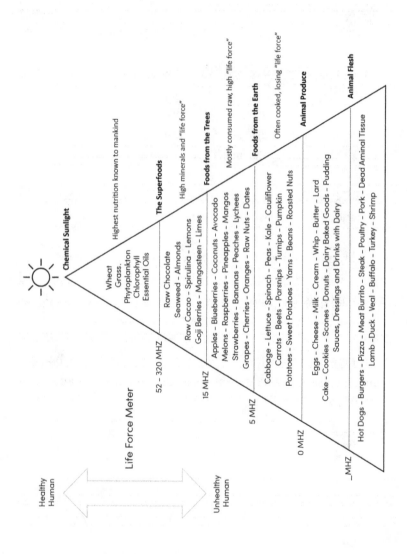

There are also many studies showing the impact of healthy food, particularly raw food, in healing chronic and deadly diseases. That is because the presence of higher, faster energy always dissolves and converts lower, slower energy. However, this is by no means intended to replace medical advice and always consult with a doctor before doing anything.

It is worth noting that you may have positive beliefs around the impact of food on your body. For example, you may have a belief within you that your body remains in a high vibration regardless of what you eat and, therefore, your physical body will always reflect those inner beliefs as with everything else in your physical reality.

That said, as your vibration rises, you will be more prone to eating healthier food as it is more energetically resonant with your general vibration and it will feel very natural to you.

Aromatherapy. Essential oils, which are made of plants, seeds, barks and flowers, are frequency elevators and their highly potent botanical properties have the capacity to lift up the frequency of the human body to match their frequency. As mentioned above, the average healthy human body vibrates at a frequency of about 70 MHz while a therapeutic-grade oil vibrates at 322 MHz (rose oil), 118 MHz (lavender) and 96 MHz (sandalwood). By inhaling or applying essential oils to the physical body, you can help raise your physical body's energetic frequency.

"Clinical research shows that essential oils have the highest frequency of any natural substance known to man, creating an

environment in which disease, bacteria, virus, fungus, etc. cannot live. I believe that the chemistry and frequencies of essential oils have the ability to help man maintain the optimal frequency to the extent that disease cannot exit."

— Gary Young of Young Living Essential Oils

However, it's important to note that not all essential oils are created equal and their quality depends on the extraction process. For aromatherapy and health purposes, it is recommended to purchase those of therapeutic grade, which is the highest quality.

I know friends who have used aromatherapy to heal anxiety and sleep better. I personally have used essential oils for boosting my mood, focusing better and relieving stomach aches. However, this is not medical advice so always consult with a doctor first.

Exercise. Needless to say that exercise helps raise your vibrational frequency, mostly because it releases endorphins, which can lower symptoms of anxiety and depression. Any time I have personally maintained an exercise routine, I have been more easily able to maintain a very high vibration.

Feng Shui. Originating from ancient China, Feng Shui is a traditional practice that uses energy forces to harmonize individuals with their environment. When you perform Feng Shui in your living and work environment, you are essentially arranging your space in such a way that maximizes the flow of energy and, therefore, attracting a multitude of enhancements for various life areas, including your relationships, health, and wealth. As with diet, when your vibration rises, you are intuitively more prone to improve the energy flow in your environment, whether you are conscious of it or not.

I recall I did Feng Shui to my bedroom many years ago when I lived with my family in Beirut. I reorganized the furniture for better flow of energy, used sea salt to clear up the energy in the dense corners of the room, and used a variety of other techniques to help shift the energy in my room. I never kept track of what happened afterwards, but I recall my best friend, Raya, reminding me of all the experiences that had taken place in my life after I did the Feng Shui, including changing jobs and moving to Dubai.

2. Emotional:
   The emotional energetic layer is where your feelings and fears reside. This is the layer that is impacted by your subconscious beliefs as well as your emotional reactions to the physical environment.

   The emotional layer is very important because emotion magnetizes thought and it is through emotions that your thoughts (both positive and negative) get imprinted as beliefs into your subconscious mind.

   The more you stabilize your feelings and emotions, the more balanced this layer will be. We spoke in Chapter 3 about the emotional vibrational scale. Each of these emotions has its frequency. As you improve your emotions, you are helping raise your own vibration.

   There are different ways to help balance your emotions, including various types of healing modalities (such as energy healing, chakra healing, crystal healing, and sound healing), meditation and breathwork, acupuncture, and, of course, traditional therapy.

Some types of music have healing properties and can help address certain emotions and raise your vibration. These include the following:

- 396-hertz frequency reduces fear and releases guilt.
- 417-hertz frequency helps dissolve negative energy and deflate the impact of sudden alterations.
- 528-hertz frequency aids miracles and transformations.
- 639-hertz frequency is suitable for building healthy relationships.
- 741-hertz frequency helps in making better decisions and finding a solution.
- 852-hertz frequency aids in spiritual orders.

I've personally used meditations and sound frequencies when my emotions were unsettled, and they've always helped me immensely.

(Disclaimer about the next section: What I share below is just an option. Not a recommendation. Always consult a doctor before taking any medication or choosing a treatment.)

For extreme emotional cases, such as anxiety and depression, traditional prescription medicine may be required. Not everyone agrees with that, but it all boils down to your core beliefs. There are also many traditional healing options mentioned above. Give yourself permission to do anything you believe will get you back on your feet.

3. Thoughts:
   Your thoughts are an extremely high frequency of pulsation that is higher than the speed of both light and sound. The frequency of thoughts can be measured, including the impact they have on your body.

   We will be talking about practiced thoughts (i.e. beliefs) in Chapter 10. However, for now, it is important to understand the impact that our thoughts have on our emotions. Our positive thoughts generate positive emotions, while our negative thoughts generate negative emotions. The thoughts are the electrical charge while the emotions are the magnetic charge. When the two come together, we create an electromagnetic field that draws in (or tunes into) a reality of similar vibration.

   That is why it is crucial to either (a) quiet the mind; or (b) practice thinking positive thoughts. Although our subconscious beliefs always supersede our conscious thoughts, our active conscious thoughts impact our emotions, which, if strong enough (positive or negative), have the power to imprint into our subconscious mind and impact the projection of our physical reality.

   Some of the same techniques used for balancing our emotions can be used to quiet the mind. These include mindfulness exercises, breathing and meditation.

4. Energy of spirit:
   The energy of spirit is the highest and fastest energy in the universe. It is the frequency of your soul, which is so incredibly rapid

that it is impossible to have any negative energy, disharmony or disease at that frequency. This is the energy stream you came from and you always have the ability to align with it by raising your vibration through meditation, and any of the above-mentioned solutions (healing, essential oils, and diet).

The one point I want to make here is that when you are following your joy, the things you need to help raise your vibration will come to you. You will not need to plan out anything or exert any effort with all the above. If you're feeling emotionally unsettled, you may be tempted to open YouTube and you'll come across an audio meditation by chance that will be exactly what you need in that moment. I cannot tell you how many times that has happened with me. Use this information as knowledge on what's out there, but let your higher mind bring you what you need in any given moment. It will be what's best for you in that circumstance.

--⇒◉ ◉⇐--

Higher consciousness means becoming aware that there is more to us than our physical conscious mind. It is an understanding that there is an inner non-physical infinite intelligence within us that has massive creative capacity, and it is guiding us every step of the way. The more you relax into that knowledge, the more you will use the higher, conscious, and subconscious minds for their intended purposes and experience magical results in the process.

PART 2

The Steps

CHAPTER 6

Intend and Imprint

Ready, Set, Create

⊶⭤ ⭢⊷

"Imagination is everything. It is the preview of life's coming attractions."

— Albert Einstein

Now that we've covered the foundations of who you are (an infinite being and creator with a signature essence) and how manifestation happens through you by projecting your physical reality outward through your subconscious mind, we can now dive into the steps of living it all.

The first step is conscious intention. It is the step that signals the green light to the universe that you are ready to step up your game and align with your core frequency – if you haven't already. This is not to say that you need to give the universe permission, since your higher mind, which is you, already knows what your highest truth is and has been guiding you at every step since your birth.

It is an important step, nevertheless, that highlights the next phase on your journey whereby you are consciously choosing to align with your purpose and highest joy.

But, first, let's explain what is meant by intention, for it is very different from goals or aspirations. In his book, *The Power of Intention*, Dr. Wayne Dyer describes intention as not being the "work of a determined ego or individual will." Intentions are not goals that you set out to do. Rather, intentions are a force that you access from an invisible source of energy (i.e. the quantum field) that has the power to take you where you need to go to live in authenticity with your higher purpose. Everything seems to "conspire" to keep you on your path. It does not require any individual willpower or physical effort on your part.

In fact, you need not even set any intentions, for that is automatically and inherently being done by your higher mind as you experience life and consciously and unconsciously identify your preferences. However, our human nature needs to have a sense of direction, and bringing intentions to our physical conscious mind's awareness helps us feel better knowing that we are moving towards a preferable destination.

Setting intentions also helps us raise our vibration, if done in the right way. It helps us experience emotions tied to the state of being of the manifested intention – essentially, living in the end state as we're setting those intentions. The emotions are a key component, for intention or thought (the electrical charge) plus emotion (the magnetic charge) together are required to imprint that intention into the subconscious mind, which then projects it out into our physical experience.

What's important in this exercise is not the actual intention set but the state of being that is achieved in the process of setting the intention that helps with the manifestation of that intention/scenario.

> I once attended an intention-setting workshop that helped me create a vision for my life and set intentions in every life area. The exercise allowed me to think about where I stood in every area of my life and what I wanted for that area. Aside from the fact that the vast majority of my intentions subsequently manifested with great ease (which I came to realize after I went back and reviewed my intentions), the exercise itself was so thrilling that it helped me significantly raise my vibration in the process. It helped me determine who I preferred to be and align with that higher and more ideal image of myself. Everything that transpired and flowed into my life from that state was the result of setting those intentions.

Ultimately, it's neither the intention itself nor the image of the ideal scenario, which you created, that matters. It's how you felt in the moment of creating those intentions and images. That raised vibration – resulting from the excitement and sense of knowing that this is who you truly are – is what is needed. Your emotions help open up your imagination to what's truly possible (if you let go of the "how"), and in doing so, you allow your higher mind to guide you on the path of manifestation of your images and scenarios in their highest form.

Your physical conscious mind has limited ability to conjure the most ideal image of any given intention (without feeling uncomfortable). That's why the role of the conscious physical mind ends with the setting of the intention. The key is to not try to involve the conscious mind in the actual creation process in any shape or form. Your goal and purpose after setting the intentions is to just forget about them.

By following the formula in Chapter 7, you allow your higher mind to guide you by opening up the path to many more possibilities and probabilities about how the actual intention could manifest.

As Bashar puts it, the ideal scenario for the physical mind is the worst scenario for the higher mind.

> For example, someone's intention may be to become the number one photographer in the country. That's what his physical conscious mind could come up with and feel good about. Stretching it further would have been uncomfortable. By basking in that feeling, and then letting it go and allowing the higher mind to guide him, he allows the manifestation to happen in the best possible way and in its highest form, which could be for him to become the number one photographer in the region or the world!
>
> His higher mind may take him on a journey that may make it seem like he's going off-path, for example, by offering him a lower-paying photography gig in another country. If he was attached to being number one in

this one particular country, and he was also focused on the money, he may turn down that opportunity. But since his higher mind has greater perspective and vision, and that is to make him number one in the region or the world, it is bringing him the opportunity that will be the gateway to make that happen.

The key is to let go of the image that was created by your physical mind and to even let go of what this whole opportunity is all about and go with the flow. *If it's exciting*, then it's a cue from the higher mind to take action on it. The higher mind is YOU and knows what you prefer and do not prefer. It will not bring to you the ultimate scenario that you would not prefer. You are the only one who would get in the way of you.

This is actually what happened with Huda Kattan, who has built a massively successful beauty empire. Her goal, as mentioned in *Gulf Business*, was to be the number-one beauty blogger in the region. Little did she know that she would by far surpass that intention and become the number-one beauty blogger in the world, with almost 50 million followers on Instagram alone.

Another example would be a woman imagining that her ex comes back to her after yet another breakup. Her physical conscious mind can imagine a scenario where her ex comes back with an apology and a desire for reconciliation. She believes that can happen because it has happened in the past. By feeling good about that and then letting it go, her higher mind can do the work.

If she truly lets go, and shuts down her physical mind's need for force or manipulation, her higher mind can help her manifest the ex back in his highest form. She may find excitement in working with a coach or taking up meditation or attending a healing retreat to unknowingly address some underlying limiting beliefs about self-worth. In following her excitement, she can raise her self-concept into a higher version of herself that is more aligned with who she really is. In that raised state – where she almost forgets about her ex – she attracts a higher version of him, whereby he comes forth with a commitment and not just another short-lived apology.

Shift Away from "Wanting" to "Preferring" or "Being"

Although I have used the word "want" frequently throughout this book for the purpose of delivering the message, when it comes to manifesting, it is important to never use the word "want." Everything is happening now. By saying "I want something," you are declaring that you don't have it and you keep yourself in that wanting space. It is crucial that you eliminate that word from your dictionary when it comes to manifesting (and anything for that matter). Want equals lack. It means "I don't have."

For example, you might say, "I want to pursue my passion for a living." Guess what? That's what you will create. Wanting to express your passion and never having that. When setting intentions, it's best to state: "My preference is to pursue my passion for a living." Or even better, state it in the present tense: "I am expressing my passion for a living." Your subconscious mind does not know that this is not already the case.

Therefore, replace the word "want" with "prefer." A preference, which is a non-judgmental neutral state, has less resistance and attachment and is simply a recognition of what is and isn't vibrationally compatible with you. It also does not indicate that something isn't there. I can prefer something I already have.

Imprinting the Intention

The key component of imprinting the intention into your subconscious mind (so that it is stored and saved) is to use emotion. You can think of the emotion as the "save" button for your thoughts so they can turn into beliefs within your subconscious mind. There is an actual science behind this.

Dr. Joe Dispenza, who is an expert on change, as well as the brain, mind and human potential, has conducted scientific research on what happens physiologically when we visualize. According to the findings, as you experience feelings and emotions while imagining your desire, oxytocin starts to be released in the brain and the heart, which signals for even more chemicals to be released in your body, causing your heart and arteries to physically and literally expand. As you do this, and you're fully in the present, the heart releases an electromagnetic field up to three meters wide. The heart, which has its own intelligence and awareness, becomes your magnet and the center of creation. That energy is frequency, and frequency carries information, which is then fed into and stored within the subconscious mind.

The options shared below for imprinting your intentions all work and are very powerful. I have used every one of these options and they are all magical. I suggest you do the same, and see which option works best for you.

These can be used for manifesting one thing or your entire new life. For the reasons mentioned earlier, every one of these options requires the use of emotions as you visualize. They are not so different from one another. They all have the same end goal and that is to have you experience – through visualization and imagination – the new reality that you prefer. What differs is how you access that state. In addition, some techniques allow the visualization to be inspired rather than initiated by you.

I do not list these in order of preference. In fact, the last one is probably my favorite because it cannot get any easier than that, and it has the least amount of attachment involved and allows your higher mind to guide you to your manifestation in its highest form.

Option 1: Neville Goddard's Method (Living in the End State)

This is probably one of the simplest methods that allows you to manifest a specific situation or experience. It is Neville Goddard's method of living in the end state, as if you already have the manifestation.

Here are the steps:

a. **Choose your intention**. The first step is to decide what your intention is. For example, your preference might be to move to another country, but you don't know how you can make that happen. Perhaps you don't have the visa requirements to live there, or you don't have a job that allows you to move, or you don't have the funds. The point is that your intention is to move. Since I love the South of France, I will use that as an example.

b. **Determine the end state**. This step requires some mental planning. Now that you have decided on your intention, think of an "end state" that would be confirmation to you that your intention has manifested. Here, it's crucial that you think of an end state that *confirms* that your intention has fully manifested.

> In the France example, the end state would be me LIVING in the South of France. I would have to make sure that the living part is clear in my end state so that I do not just manifest a visit or vacation. I may come up with an end state where I am signing a long-term lease on an apartment in France or I experience myself talking with a friend and informing them that I have moved to the South of France.

c. **Plant the seed**. Once you've determined what your end state is, as you're going to sleep, visualize it with utmost clarity and with the emotions involved in living that end state. The best way to do that is to activate your five senses so you feel what it would be like to be living in that end state. Let your emotions go there fully.

But the caveat is this. You must visualize yourself living that end state in the first person and not in the third person. For example, I may visualize a scene where, as an outside observer, I see myself signing the long-term lease on an apartment in France. That would be visualizing in third-person point of view and should never be visualized as the end state. Instead, I visualize myself – in the first person – as I am signing the long-term lease on the apartment. Otherwise, you might manifest someone else doing that while you're simply the observer. Remember, the subconscious mind doesn't know "what you mean." It has no analytical capabilities. It projects what you feed it and will reproduce a scene where you are observing, not signing.

For best results, it is highly recommended that you plant the seed right as you're going to sleep when your active analytical mind has shut down. As your brain waves slow down, any visualizations will be imprinted faster into your subconscious mind. Visualize the end state in its entirety while feeling the emotion of living it. Keep doing that until you fall asleep. With this step, you will plant the seed into your subconscious mind.

d. **Let it go.** This step will be the same for every option I provide in this section. Your active role ends here. The next step will be to follow your excitement (Chapter 7).

With this option, once you've planted the seed for a given intention, you really should not go back and plant another seed for the same intention. You may be tempted to fill the gap between where you are now and the end state by "visualizing the middle." Remember, your physical mind has no idea how the middle part will play out. By trying to visualize the middle, you are trying to take control with your physical mind. The higher mind (and only your higher mind) has that perspective. So let go of HOW this will happen. Do not visualize the middle. I say this because I have been tempted to do that many times.

In the France example, I may be tempted to visualize myself manifesting a job (and, therefore, a "work permit") that will allow me to move there. If my end goal is France (and not necessarily the job), I should not try to fill in the middle part with options I think will get me there. There might be a much higher form of the manifestation for me that allows me to remain self-employed (which is something I prefer) AND live in France. Your higher mind knows everything that you prefer and will bring you your manifestation in its highest form.

Here's another example. Let's say you want to manifest marriage to an ideal partner. So your end state would be visualizing yourself with a partner and celebrating your one-year wedding anniversary. This would be a definite full manifestation of your desire. Then, at some point, you feel tempted to imagine a "middle stage" such as how you meet that person. The problem with this is that you are trying to use your physical mind to control how it plays out. You

> have no idea how the middle will play out and you
> may actually manifest meeting someone in the exact
> way you imagined but they are not the one you will
> marry. So you will be completely disappointed once
> your end state does not manifest. Focus on the end
> and let go of the middle.

You also do not want to be tempted to change the end state to accommodate your limiting beliefs. That's why the key is to plan it out (step b) before planting the seed (step c).

Finally, do not remain in visualization. Once you plant the seed, let it go. There is a huge reason why I highly recommend this and it's because by constantly remaining in the visualization, you are at risk of feeling the lack of it in your present reality. You also do not want to miss living in the present moment, which is where your life is now and where you can live many joyful experiences, as your higher mind works in the background to bring to you your manifestation.

I've done this. I've spent too much time visualizing, almost to the point where I was no longer in the present and was, instead, living in the future. This is not what we want here. Our lives are now, and it's always about the journey of creation, not the destination.

Option 2: The Pure Technique

If you have an inspired desire within you, it means that a version of you is already living it in a parallel reality and you have the full potential to live that reality too. You've tapped into that reality through your higher mind and that's how the desire is inspired within you.

In his book *Parallel Universes of Self,* Frederick Dodson shares a powerful technique called "The Pure Technique" that allows you to tap into a parallel reality where a version of you is already living that reality. Essentially, it is surfing through actual parallel realities.

Do keep an open mind. I promise, if you do, you will experience this process in a truly magical way.

The steps are as follows:

a. **Define an intention you would like to experience**. In the same way we did in option 1, decide what intention you would like to experience. If you do not have any particular intention in mind, think about something non-preferred in your current life (such as a draining job) and request to experience the opposite of that.

> Going back to my South of France example, my intention could be something like this: "I would like to experience a reality in which I am living in the South of France."

Notice here, we did not determine a scenario that would confirm manifestation of the end state as we did in option 1. We kept it open but clear. Also, notice that I did not say "permanently living." Unless you are absolutely sure, you want to try to remain fluid in your intentions because you don't know how you will feel after a few years of living there. You may want to change perspectives and move somewhere else. So allow yourself to be flexible, albeit clear about what you don't want. In my case, I'm clear that I'm living there and not just visiting.

This option would also be fantastic for experiencing a future reality where you are living your highest potential. This would bring you into a vision of your whole life and not just the experience of one intention.

b. **Relax into zero point (be silent).** In this step, you want to get into a neutral observer mode.

To do that, close your eyes and focus on quieting your mind. You want to go into a zero point, which is a thoughtless state. Forget about the outside world. Forget about your desire as well as any problems you may be facing. Forget about what you're going to have for lunch. Forget it all.

This may require practice because our minds tend to run on autopilot. The best way to quiet your mind is to focus on your breathing. Notice how you breathe in and then breathe out, then breathe in again and breathe out. Keep focusing on your breath in every moment. By doing that, you relax into your body and you quiet your mind. You will start to feel yourself drifting into a void of nothingness, with no sensation of your body. Keep yourself in that observation mode as you become aware of that inner presence within you.

Once you achieve that state (which may take from a few minutes to 20 minutes or even more), you are now at zero point. Allow that space to be created.

c. **Allow the "vision" to come in**. In this step, allow yourself to receive an image of a version of yourself living that experience. This is slightly different from visualization because it is coming to you without effort, whereas in visualization, you are coming up with the image using your mind (as you did in option 1).

In this case, the image is coming to you. Observe it. See what's going on. Check out who's there. In this step, you are the observer just looking into the scene. This is a crucial step because you are literally tapping into an actual parallel reality. This already exists and a version of you is already living it.

> In my France example, I did this exercise and came into a beautiful property overlooking the bay of Villefranche-sur-Mer, which is a picturesque location in the South of France, and I saw a version of myself and my entire family there enjoying a lunch gathering on the terrace, with my nieces playing in the pool with their friends.

Allow yourself to do the same and take in the whole scene. But since we are an observer in this step, we cannot stay here. When you feel you have captured enough of the scene, you need to move to the next step, where you actually *enter the viewpoint of that version of you*.

d. **Enter the viewpoint**. So here, instead of looking AT that version of ourselves, we enter the viewpoint of this person who is already experiencing complete fulfillment of that desired reality. So we are becoming them.

As that person, experience that reality fully and experience the joy, natural ease, gratitude, and happiness of living that moment. Do not experience it just as a mental event. Live it and experience the full body sensations of that experience in terms of sight, sounds, scents, touch, and taste. When you do this, the emotions within you will be activated.

> So in my example, I am now experiencing the viewpoint of that person in the family gathering. I *hear* the sounds of the girls playing and splashing in the pool, I *feel* the warmth of the sun on my skin, I *look* at and take in the stunning view of the bay, I *smell* the salty air of the Mediterranean, and I *taste* the freshly squeezed lemonade I just prepared for the family. I *hear* the laughter and joy of the family.

Can you see how your emotions are activated with this full-body experience? Don't do this in order to experience it later. Live it now and experience the joy of it right here and right now.

Rest in that space for a few minutes before releasing it and opening your eyes.

e. **Let it go**. In the hours, days and weeks after, simply rest in the fulfillment of that desire, and you do that by just letting it go. Don't think about it. Don't affirm or visualize any further. Don't try to make anything happen. Drop it. In fact, forget it.

As with option 1, life continues as usual, and you'll follow your excitement in every moment, as we'll cover later.

Option 3: The Essence of What I Want

If you are someone who is not clear about what you want and you have not been able to create an image of where you would like to go, this technique would be perfect for you.

In fact, this technique is highly recommended because there is no attachment involved to any mental image or intention and, therefore, you are giving yourself the full flexibility to just go with the flow.

In this technique, you focus only on the essence of what you'd like to experience in every area of your life.

Below are some examples. They are essentially a list of values that you may have for each category and that are important to you. In the examples below, these values are defined with words. The key here is to FEEL the essence of everything you are listing because that is what will anchor them into your subconscious mind. It's also important to think of what you definitely don't want and then write the opposite. Beware to not write down anything that you do not want because you do not want to imprint that into your subconscious mind.

Career	Finances
Passion	Freedom
Flexible working hours	Well-being
Creativity	Divine support
Ease	Abundance
Fun	Ease
Freedom	Flow
Friendly and relaxed environment	Liquidity
Success	Growth in wealth
Growth	Debt-free
Small team	
Family atmosphere	
Romantic Relationship	**Family**
Mutual love	Quality time
Equal love	Fun and adventure
Passion	Laughter
Respect and understanding	Love
Fun and laughter	Compassion
Joy	Respect
Commitment	
Long-term	
Two-way attraction	
Soulmate who is single (This would be the opposite of married as you do not want to attract someone who is married)	

Physical Body	State of Being
Healthy	Happy
Radiant	Joyful
Youthful	Fulfilled
Fit and toned	Relaxed
Active	At ease
Vibrant	In flow
	Feeling good
	Graceful
	Empowered

As a final word here: let the whole point of all these exercises be for the purpose of feeling extremely excited and passionate about your new life. Then just let it go.

I cannot emphasize how important the letting go part is because when you remain too focused on it, you're trying too hard. Insistence creates resistance.

Let it go.

CHAPTER 7

Stay Present and Follow Your Joy

It's All About the Journey, Not the Destination

⊷▄ ◉ ▄⊶

"Happiness is the meaning and the purpose of life, the whole aim and end of human existence."

— Aristotle

In her book *Dying to Be Me*, Anita Moorjani shares details about her near-death experience and her brief encounter with the non-physical world. It is a book that I highly recommend you read, for it brings a great deal of insight into how the non-physical world functions.

In the short time she was in the spiritual world, she experienced instant manifestation. She would think a thought, and she'd automatically experience the manifestation of it. This is how manifestations take place in the non-physical. In the physical world, the illusion of time creates a time lag, which is sometimes very brief, between the setting of an intention and its manifestation. This allows us to experience the process of creation, which is how we agreed to experience the physical world in order to learn about our creative abilities and to experience the unfolding. The time lag also allows us to fine-tune our intentions and/or change our minds!

This chapter is all about the unfolding of our manifestations with regards to the intentions we imprinted in our subconscious minds through the processes described in the previous chapter.

Hopefully, by now, you have already imprinted some intentions. If not, I highly recommend you stop and do this now. Knowledge is power, but true knowledge comes from experience, and you will not truly grasp the concepts I am sharing here unless you actually go through the steps yourself.

After you've set and imprinted your intentions, your goal is to let go and forget about the intentions. As you do this, you will start to feel a tug or a sense of excitement urging you to take certain actions. This sense of excitement may feel random and the actions may seem totally unrelated to the intentions you've set.

Your goal is to not question or wonder why you feel excited about a certain action. Just drop your physical mind's need to overanalyze, go with the flow, and follow your joy in every moment.

The formula, provided in the teachings of Bashar, specifically states the following:

1. Act on your highest excitement
2. To the best of your ability

3. With zero assumption or insistence on what the outcome is supposed to look like
4. And remain in a positive state no matter what the outcome is in order to derive the full benefit

Act on Your Highest Excitement

The first step in the formula is to act on your highest sense of excitement or joy.

Your higher mind sends a "signal" to your physical mind that can be interpreted as the feeling of excitement or passion in your body. By acting on this excitement, you are allowing your higher mind to guide you towards the manifestation of your intentions.

As Bashar defines it, "Excitement is the energy that occurs when one is in resonance with their own Higher Self. This is a 'signal' from your Higher Self (which always honors your free will) to encourage you to act or move in a particular direction. Excitement can therefore be used as a 'compass heading' to move and act in the direction that your Higher Self hopes you will move – for your highest joy. If you follow your excitement consistently, you will end up fulfilling your Life's Purpose."

The key word here is the "highest" excitement. This means choosing an action that has more excitement, passion, curiosity, attractiveness, or love than any other choice at a particular moment. This could be as small and ordinary as having coffee with a friend, going to the mall, or taking a walk or it could be as big and life-spanning as starting a new business, moving to a new country, getting a new degree, or quitting your existing job.

The actions themselves may not seem tied to your intentions, but that is not for your physical mind to think or wonder about. They are actions that are taking you somewhere towards fulfilling your dreams.

As you start following your sense of excitement or passion in every moment, you will start building momentum as your higher mind starts to bring you even more opportunities to get excited about.

When you feel passionate or drawn to more than one action or opportunity at a particular moment, take action on the one that brings the higher level of excitement, even if just by a tiny bit. So, for example, if you are excited about both going to the mall and having coffee with a friend, choose the option that excites you more, even if the difference appears very slight.

The key is to ACT, for "action is the language of physical reality."

It is not enough to feel excited. You should take action on that passion. Following your joy is not being excited about wanting something. It should be about HAVING something, and that requires taking action. Otherwise, there will be no purpose for your higher mind to send you more opportunities because you are not taking action.

In addition, the excitement may often build up within you, and if you do not take action, it may show up physically in your body through pains and aches.

This is exactly what happened to me when I felt the urge to shift into coaching but did not take action. Six years after growing my first business regionally, and building a large online presence, I felt a high sense of urgency to shift into coaching. It was something I had wanted for some time, and it was definitely part of my excitement. But I did not take action immediately, despite my eagerness and excitement to do so.

Looking back, I now know that I had limiting beliefs holding me back. As the weeks passed, I felt the build-up of energy in my body and started to experience intense and chronic migraines. As these headaches persisted, they were becoming quite debilitating. My intuition (higher mind) told me that this was due to lack of action on my calling. But I still went to see a doctor anyway, and he prescribed a CT scan, with a follow-up appointment scheduled for the following week.

Meanwhile, over the weekend, as I opened up my laptop, I felt a surge of energy flowing through me. Before I knew what hit me, I had created the website, logo, and marketing message for my new business. I used that logo for seven years, and I was complimented on it by a graphic designer. I still don't know how I did it. It usually takes me days and sometimes weeks to "get things right." Not in this case. Everything just flowed, and in 24 hours, I had fully established my coaching business.

> I was so mesmerized by the whole process that I did not even realize that my headache was gone for the first time in four weeks. And it never came back. On the insistence of my dear mother, I still went to see the doctor for the follow-up appointment to discuss the results of the CT scans. I smiled and was grateful when the doctor confirmed that my scans were "just perfect," to use his exact words. Even his words were no accident.

The key is to take action, as best as you can for as long as you can.

If, at some point, you feel your excitement waning – provided you are not making that happen with your own limiting beliefs and definitions – then it may be time to search for the next option that contains higher excitement than any other choice.

Is Your Excitement Waning or Is Your Physical Mind Interjecting?

You have to be careful not to confuse the waning of excitement with an interjection by your physical mind. For example, you may start to wonder where all these actions are taking you. Your mind may not be able to figure out the purpose of these actions and you may start to question if you're on the right path. You might feel compelled to stop the momentum because you can't see where it's going or you're doubting the process.

Remain conscious and aware of your physical mind's need to take control of the steering wheel.

To the Best of Your Ability

The next step in the formula is to keep taking action on your excitement for as far as you can until you can take it no further. Any action that would involve you not abiding by the laws and/or rules/ethics of society is a signal that you can't take it further. This is a physical limitation that is clearly informing you that the road straight ahead is no longer your path. That is when you must stop and search for an alternate route.

> For example, in following your excitement, you decide to create an animal shelter to care for stray dogs and cats. Let's say that within the laws of the country where you would like to set up the shelter, you are required to get a permit from the municipality or a similar government authority. Yet despite your best efforts, you are not granted the permit. This would be an example of a physical limitation, and you must search for an alternate route, which may not require a permit, such as finding foster families to help care for the animals in their own homes. Or, simply, if you can't find an alternate route, it's a sign that you need to let it go, if you have genuinely pursued it to the best of your ability.

The point is to not get out of alignment when you come up against physical limitations such as these, for this might be a signal for you that it is time to stop or shift directions.

With Zero Assumption and Insistence on Outcome

The third step in the formula is to act on your highest excitement with *zero assumption and insistence on what the outcome is supposed to look like.* This is because your physical mind does not know what the best possible outcome needs to look like.

By insisting on a particular outcome, you are actually placing limits on what the ideal outcome could be, and that outcome may be many times better than what your physical mind is capable of imagining. Therefore, it is important to remain humble enough to let go of the idea that your physical mind knows for certain what the best outcome may be for you. But your higher mind does because it has a higher perspective.

> For example, if you would like to attract a romantic partner, and you feel excited about attending a party, your physical mind might jump to the conclusion that you're going to meet someone at the party. So when you attend the party and do not meet anyone, you might feel disappointed and wonder "what went wrong?" or "why do things not work out for me?" The key is to not jump to any conclusions or have expectations about why you feel excited about attending a party. You don't know what's in this for you. You should be excited just for feeling excited without concluding that this might be leading you to a specific desire. It might be that you will meet

someone who might eventually introduce you to someone or you might build a new work-related connection that can get you a new job, which may also be
related to another intention you have set.

Or, simply, the party is intended to allow you to just have
fun, which is a way to raise your vibration and keep your
mind off your desire! That may be the only reason!

Sometimes, the form of excitement comes in a way that will get you
to act because your higher mind knows that if it comes to you in that
form, you will take action on it, and then it can lead you to where you
need to be so that what really needs to happen, can happen for you.

Choose to Remain in a Positive State No Matter What the Outcome Is In Order to Derive the Full Benefit

The previous step highlighted that there should be zero insistence on
what the outcome should be. This means that when an outcome manifests that is objectively not an outcome you would prefer, then it is very
important to remain in a positive state.

There are no accidents. This is an outcome that you need to experience in that moment and it must have happened for a purpose that
will serve you. By remaining positive, you will be able to see why that
showed up and extract the benefit from it.

In the previous chapter, I gave the example of a photographer, who has set the intention to become the number-one photographer in his country. But he has some limiting unconscious beliefs that do not support his intention. As part of his excitement, he meets a fantastic new customer, who quickly decides to work with him. It's all flowing with synchronicity in a wonderful way until the customer shows up one day extremely unhappy and criticizes all the work delivered. The photographer may get confused and wonder how and why he attracted this "negative" situation even though he's been following his excitement every step of the way.

This would be an example of when the photographer should remain in a positive space in order to derive the full benefit from this outcome. He asks himself, "What would I have to believe about myself in order to have attracted this outcome?"

After some thought, he realizes that he may have some subconscious limiting beliefs about his photographic abilities as a result of someone ridiculing his photography when he was young and just starting out. He was not aware that he's holding on to this, but through this outcome, he was able to bring this belief to his conscious awareness. The minute he does, he is able to release that negative belief and even manifest a positive outcome with the same client.

Meanwhile, the key is to never give up or think that you can't manifest or you're doing something wrong. Most importantly, never take yourself out of alignment as a result of an outcome that you do not prefer (in this example, the unhappy client). It happened for a very good reason. It's all part of bringing you the ultimate manifestation in its highest form.

When you learn to trust the process and stay in a positive place regardless of what's happening, you will not only derive the full benefit (in this case, releasing the limiting belief), but you will also unlock the seven elements of excitement, which we will cover in the next chapter.

What If You're at Work All Day?

People are prone to find excuses for why this formula may not work for them. If you are at work all day, how can you possibly follow your excitement?

There are no barriers to divine orchestration. You have to know that – even while you're at work – synchronicities will organize your day to the last minute, even with your boss watching over you.

A few years ago, I worked on a high-pressure consulting project that took up my entire work schedule. I had a very clear intention and that was to experience ease and flow in any given day and to work on what I wanted when I wanted. I cannot tell you how perfectly synchronized my days often were without ever having to force anything. Meetings I didn't feel like attending would get rescheduled on the request of someone else. People would come late to a meeting, giving me just enough time to complete a task on my to-do list. Deadlines would be extended on the request of another person, giving me more time to complete the task on time. And so on.

Remain open and trust that everything will flow in the way it should regardless of how busy you are.

Even Your Chores Can Feel Joyful

We all have chores that we may have to do that we don't particularly enjoy doing, such as cleaning our home, doing the laundry, going to the grocery store and any other various chores that are not fun.

As you follow your joy, everything you need to do becomes so easy and you actually feel excited about doing some of these tasks, believe it or not!

The formula and synchronicity will apply to every single detail in your life, including your chores. You suddenly feel the urge to do these random chores and they will fit perfectly into your day. They will not feel like chores, and you'll find yourself enjoying them somehow.

This flow and synchronicity applies to every area.

Remain open and do not let your physical mind convince you that this will not work for you. It works for everyone, every time. No exceptions.

⋅►▌══◉ ◉══▐◄⋅

The beauty of this formula is that it's automatically helping you raise your practiced vibration. There's no "pre-work" that you need to do in order to get started. You start right away by doing the things you love to do and this helps you raise your vibration.

It is also a tool that helps a person stay present without thinking too much about what they want, as that may take them into a place of lack.

CHAPTER 8

Ride the Wave

Synchronicities, Abundance and Flow

-+≡⊙ ⊙≡+-

When you follow the four-step formula of the previous chapter, you
unlock the seven elements of excitement. As Bashar puts it, "your life
will become an ecstatic explosion of synchronicity and will continue to
grow and expand in that way ... and your higher mind will attract to
you all the different synchronicities, opportunities, circumstances, and
situations that are of the highest form, vibration and representation of
your ideal scenario."

There will be such a momentum created that you will KNOW that
whatever comes your way is all part of the plan. You will never have to
second-guess or wonder what this is about. You will just go with the
flow, feeling the excitement every step of the way.

Essentially, as you follow the four steps of "acting on your highest
excitement to the best of your ability with no insistence on outcome
and staying in a positive state no matter what," you will unlock multiple elements of excitement and synchronicities in the following ways:

1. Your life becomes a driving engine.

    You start to feel the momentum of energy flowing through you as your excitement and passion inject you with so much energy that you can't wait to get up in the morning and take action.

2. Your life becomes an organizing principle of synchronicity.

    You will receive the things in the order that you need to act on them. You will feel which things contain more excitement and passion than any other choices so you can act on them first. It literally organizes your day. Whatever you didn't have time to act on by the end of the day when you are excited about going to sleep, you didn't need to act on that day. Every facet of your life will literally be organized, allowing you to experience a monumental flow of perfect timing in terms of how things and opportunities come to you exactly when you need them – not a moment before but not a moment later than you need them.

> During 2020, after following my excitement in writing this book, I was swept up by a wave of synchronicities – all divinely orchestrated – that would organize my day down to the minute. I would get up in the morning, not knowing what my day would look like but simply acting on the step that excited me the most in any given moment and always remaining present in that moment. I never had to guess or worry about what was next because I was going with the flow and doing what brought me the most joy in that moment.
>
> Every action was either fueling me with more energy and passion or simply assisting me in writing my book

by bringing to me all the resources or tools that would be useful, including great examples to share with my readers, writing courses to help me write, and meditation tools to help me gain further clarity.

3. Path of Least Resistance.

Your life starts to flow more effortlessly. You don't have to push anything forward or force things to happen. The path unfolds before you automatically, allowing you to flow through your life more easily, and you witness your manifestations happening effortlessly. That is because your higher mind is navigating you through your limiting subconscious beliefs so you can either easily release them or go around them. It's step by step. There are no big or uncomfortable jumps in the process.

I first decided to write this book in December 2019. I reached out to a publishing coach for help. I didn't hear back from him. I was actually working on a consulting project and was quite busy, so I didn't pursue it further. Then the coronavirus hit the world in 2020. The work on this project started to slow down in March 2020. After having worked non-stop for 2.5 years on this project, I was quite exhausted, so I took the time to just relax and unwind. I spent about a month in that space of literally not doing anything but centering myself. I did whatever helped in that regard, from painting to watching series after series on Netflix to reading. Had I attempted to pursue the book during that period, it would have been difficult. I needed to hit the reset button on myself, and this was what I needed in that moment.

In April, I decided to get clear once again on my intentions for every area of my life. Needless to say, my intentions included writing and publishing my book. The whole intention-setting exercise helped me raise my vibration and get in touch with how I saw my life unfolding. It was such a beautiful and deliberate phase, in which I got back in touch with how I wished my life to unfold. I immediately started seeing manifestations.

I did not have to force anything. The actions were inspired in the moment, and I would just do what I felt excited to do without a second thought.

One morning in May, as soon as I woke up, I remembered the book intention and thought, "I really would like to write that book." When I opened my laptop less than an hour later, I found an email in my inbox from the publishing coach I had emailed back in December. He apologized for missing my email of December and wanted to see if I still wanted to write my book. I couldn't help but smile at that synchronicity. It was all divinely timed. Of course, I signed up and started working on the book right away.

Your path will unfold in such a way that everything you want comes on the path of least resistance. You never have to put in effort or force anything. Had

I attempted to write my book back in December, it
would have felt like a difficult task. I was not in the
space to do it at that time.

4. & 5. Path of Connection and Relevance.

Your life will flow in such a way that your path will connect you to
all expressions of excitement in your life that are relevant for you
to experience: the people, places, experiences, and circumstances.
What's relevant is what is aligned with your unique frequency. All
that will come in and light up the path for you. These will be
people who may knowingly or unknowingly teach you what you
need to learn on your path or connect you to others that are important on your journey. You may manifest non-preferred experiences
that may shed light on some beliefs you are holding on to that may
not be serving you. By remaining positive and becoming aware of
these beliefs and releasing them, the path will light up further for
you, and it will become clear why and how you attracted those
experiences into your life.

The path will include everything that is relevant to you in experiencing the manifestation of your intentions in their highest forms
so you achieve your intentions in the most fulfilling way.

Whatever intentions you may have set that do not manifest will
not be relevant, at least not for now. But you will not care because
you will be experiencing a magical flow of experiences that you
will not even notice what does not come and if you do, you will
not miss it because you will realize that it's not aligned with your
core frequency in that moment.

6. Path of Support

The path you're following will bring to you the form of abundance necessary for you to continue acting on your joy. The key here is to not get hung up on how this will happen.

The most important point is never to chase after abundance. As you start pursuing your passion, you may find yourself getting financially depleted (which may not necessarily happen, and it all depends on your belief systems). But let's say that happens. At times, you may be tempted to force things. To "pitch" ideas to people as an attempt to bring in the income. If you do that, you may face some resistance unless this is truly part of your excitement and not a fear-based action (you will learn to discern the difference).

You have to believe that abundance will always flow in divine timing. You never have to force it.

> I have been self-employed since 2011. My ability to remain open has allowed me to manifest different income streams. Some of them were from my own coaching business through private clients and programs; at other times, they were through consulting and training work, which has continued to flow in all these years since I left the corporate world. It was all work that I was aligned with and was fun and exciting for me to work on. With time, I have started to realize that my knowledge and skills across different areas of work (from entrepreneurship to online businesses to corporate consulting) all seem to be relevant for any new project I take on.

Your path will take you on a journey of honing your unique skills and passions so that you can apply them all very uniquely in the work you do. You will really be excited and fulfilled. I stopped trying to compartmentalize myself into one area and have just been going with the flow.

Any time I insisted that the abundance needed to come in a certain way (for example, from a program I launched or from private clients), I slowed down the momentum. When I learned to truly let go and remain appreciative of what flowed in, I was able to receive the support in the most timely fashion through various opportunities (because when there is no insistence, you open up the possibilities, and you allow synchronicity to do its work).

By the time COVID-19 hit, work slowed down for me. But I was not really impacted because I had accumulated a cushion of funds that ultimately sustained me until the end of the year. During that seven-month period, I started writing my book, invested in some courses, rebranded my business and changed the core message, and redid the entire website. This was all a prepping stage for the new path I was choosing in terms of shifting from a business coach to a spiritual coach. In that incubation period, I was investing rather than receiving. But I was fully supported because I had the funds needed to both invest in these actions and keep me going on a personal level during that time.

By December 2020, I started to sense that it was time to bring in new income. Within a few days, I received the first consulting project, which was truly fun and exciting. About a month into working on that project, which was expected to be about two months long, I received a second consulting opportunity. I found it surprising that these consulting gigs came at the same time, but I knew there must be a reason. Midway through those two, one of the projects was paused for two weeks to squeeze in yet another small project for the same client. This brought a quick and easy third income stream into the picture. Although the two projects were scheduled to end at different times, due to random events, both projects ended at exactly the same time in March 2021.

Even my friends and family noticed how synchronistic that was.

Once these projects were completed, I was on the final run of finishing my book. So, I used the time from March until May to work on that. During that writing phase, I was supported financially from all three consulting projects, which were all divinely orchestrated to support my passion in writing this book.

You truly have to live it to see how divine timing works. Let go of the fear and allow the universe to work on your behalf. When you do, you will just KNOW that you are always supported.

According to Bashar, "Abundance is the ability to do what you need to do when you need to do it." Abundance comes in different forms so be open to what comes in. Sometimes, it will not be through expressing a specific passion but will be through work you enjoy, as in my case. Remain open. You may also be offered support through an investor or a gift. Do not limit your definition of abundance, and the more you remain open, the more abundance can come to you in the way that would most benefit you.

7. Reflective Mirror Tool.

The final element on your path of excitement will be the reflective mirror tool. As you follow your joy and passion, you may manifest outcomes that are objectively not what you prefer or that are out of alignment with your passion. If that happens – and you have indeed been in a positive place and following your joy – then it means that you may have subconscious beliefs that need to be released. The manifested outcomes have manifested to bring those beliefs to light, provided you choose to remain in a positive place and not react negatively to the circumstances. Use this negative outcome as a reflective mirror to show you what is lurking in your subconscious mind so that you can release it.

When you dig in and retrieve the core belief that is behind the negative outcome, you will be able to see that it does not make sense and, consequently, will be able to release it. Once you do that, you will again add energy to the momentum (without the weight of these subconscious beliefs) and accelerate yourself even more quickly on your path.

Divine Support

Probably the biggest roadblock for people not pursuing their passions is the financial aspect. They can't see how they can do it and support themselves and their families financially.

But when you start to understand that you are a spiritual being created in the image of "source" and you are having this physical experience for the purpose of "being yourself to the best of your ability," then you will begin to have faith that you will always be supported, for that is your very purpose for existence.

If not, you wouldn't exist! Being YOU allows "source" to expand awareness of itself through the process of creation in this physical reality.

All you need to do is follow your excitement and passion and everything that you need will come to you when you need it. In the beginning, you will be acting purely on faith, but once you experience this for yourself and realize how everything comes to you exactly when you need it, you will KNOW you are always supported.

> Another perfect example I can give for divine support is that of a friend, who runs her own business. Early on in her journey of running her own business, her rental payment was due to be paid but she didn't have the full amount available. In Dubai, the weekend is Friday and Saturday. Her rent was due to be paid on a Sunday. By Thursday night, which was the end of the working week, right before the Sunday when the check was due, she did not have the funds to pay the rent.

Her rent is paid through post-dated checks so the landlord would be cashing the check on Sunday, and if there were no funds in the account, the check would bounce and she would be at risk of going to jail. She was literally at a loss of what to do until she realized that there wasn't anything she could do but surrender.

She spent most of Friday sleeping so that she wouldn't feel compelled to think and worry about it. She just let it go. By Saturday morning, keeping in mind that it was still the weekend, she got three consecutive calls from three different clients requesting her services. Just like that, she was able to pay her rent in full on the due date.

The key is to not dwell on things. She couldn't do anything but surrender.

Another great example showcasing divine support involves advice I received from a financial advisor to invest LESS than I had initially proposed. Have you ever heard of that before? A financial advisor suggesting you invest less?

Several years ago, I set an intention to manifest an abundance of liquid cash in my bank account. I don't know why I affirmed that specifically but, needless to say, it manifested. Then at one point, I felt it was too much cash just lying around like that, and as I was comfortable with a certain minimum balance, and funds were consistently coming in, I found myself over-spending. So I set a new intention to manage my funds better, for higher and longer-term returns.

As a result, about six months prior to COVID-19, I started a savings plan with the help of a financial advisor. Part of the plan required that I set aside each month – for the first 22 months – a fixed amount that I would not be able to change or withdraw. I proposed a certain amount, which the financial advisor thought about, and then proposed I go for half that amount to start with. I was surprised but certainly took his advice.

Although it was in his interest to get a higher payment blocked in, he proposed I invest half the amount. Looking back, I have no doubt in my mind that this was divinely supported because COVID-19 hit the world six months later and the contract I was on ended sooner than expected. The amount I retained in liquidity, as a result of the lower savings plan, helped support me during 2020.

As you pursue your passion, your faith may be tested at times. Persist and believe. Once you surpass that initial period of building faith and move into the KNOWING that you are supported, the abundance will flow in and you won't be bothered thinking about it.

Your physical mind can't imagine "how" you will be able to pull it off. But so long as you stay in that space of excitement and passion, you will be okay.

If you can't let the anxiety go, then you can always go to bed, as my friend did that weekend when her rent was due. Sleep stops the resistance and fear.

The key is to not try to interfere and make things happen. For example, you might feel compelled to ask someone for help (even though it doesn't feel good – so it's not coming from a place of excitement). That would be your physical mind trying to take control of the steering wheel. I certainly did that a couple of times in the beginning because I did have that option. My friend did not have that option, so all she could do was surrender. You really have to remain strong and allow this "learning phase" to pass. When you're cutting it close, know that you're being shown that the universe has your back and that you are always supported. As Bashar puts it, "you get exactly what you need when you need it, not a minute before and not a minute after."

Don't think for one minute that this is how it will always be. In the beginning, you may cut things close, like my friend did in the above example. This is part of the learning phase, so you really start to understand how this works. Once you receive the funds you need in such a timely manner, you will understand that there is divine orchestration at work. It can't be coincidence. Once you experience this, that's when you can move from just having faith to KNOWING that you are always supported.

Remember this. Abundance is always a by-product of being YOU.

Negative Synchronicities

Sometimes, when you are riding the wave of synchronicities, you will experience negative synchronicities, which are intended to stop you from going in a particular direction. This often happens when your physical mind tries to interfere.

A negative synchronicity happens when you attempt to move in a certain direction but it does not flow. It will be obvious to you when you compare it to those experiences that flow fully and easily. When you experience this "lack of flow," pay attention. It is highly likely that you are trying to interfere with the process using your physical mind and are on a path that is not yours.

The best way to understand negative synchronicity is to know what positive synchronicity is. As I was rebranding my business, I felt myself struggling with how to reposition myself (thereby unknowingly setting the intention to receive guidance and support). Soon thereafter, I randomly received a coaching video filmed by a business coach. I highly resonated with her approach and style and immediately decided to check out her coaching program, to which I applied and quickly received a positive response. I was blown away by how much value she offered for an incredibly low investment. Needless to say, low cost is also a form of abundance and support! I signed up, completed the entire online program, and applied all the work on my business, thereby receiving the full value of the course. This is an example of positive synchronicity, where the path opened up, I followed my joy in working with the coach (without too much thinking and calculation), and I derived the full benefit from the work.

A negative synchronicity is the opposite of that. Having enjoyed my work with the coach, one day, I decided to activate my physical mind and search through her other programs. There was no specific need or requirement that needed addressing in that moment. Yet, I still searched. I came across a certification program, which I had seen a few times but never felt compelled to sign up for. As I read through the program, I built up some excitement around taking this course. Looking back, I realize that it wasn't even part of my highest excitement. It was my physical mind interfering and thinking that this might be a good certification to have. When I applied, it took some time to hear back from the coach (giving me plenty of room to think about it!). When I heard back from her, I realized that the investment was quite high. It was literally five times the price of the other course, which I had needed.

I was surprised. But I decided to go for it anyway.

I invested in the course through an installment plan. And I have to say that every time the installment went through, it felt heavy. It felt expensive. And I only took a few lessons and never completed the program.

This is a perfect example of negative synchronicity. Firstly, it didn't come to me. I went searching for something (not knowing what!). Secondly, I didn't need it. It was my physical mind trying to fit a piece into the puzzle. Thirdly, it didn't flow because it took the coach several days to respond (which was unusual). Fourthly, the investment "felt" too high. In actuality, it's never about the actual amount you are paying but how you feel about it. You can be paying a very high price for something and still feel its affordability. But in this case, since it was not what I needed in that moment, I was not aligned with the pricing.

Learn to notice these types of negative synchronicities because they are a sign that this is not the path for you. This course was not relevant for me. At least, it wasn't in that moment ("path of relevance"). I also wonder if it will ever be relevant. It's not my path and I chose to force it using my physical mind.

When the path is yours, it will unfold before you and come to you in perfect timing and in an optimal package.

⋅→▸━◉ ◉━◂←⋅

When you unlock the elements of excitement and synchronicities, you will literally feel yourself riding a wave of excitement, support, and synchronicities. Everything you receive feels incredibly timely, such as the publishing coach responding to me in the exact moment I remembered my intention. He unknowingly reached out when I was ready.

Everything that comes your way is synchronistic, just like the low-investment business coaching program that I needed and came to me randomly and which I signed up for and completed in full.

Everything that is relevant will come to you. You will not have to search for anything. But it's still okay if you do because negative synchronicity will come into the picture and show you that something is not relevant and part of your path at this moment. Learn to notice the difference. When something does not flow, it is not your path. At least, not now. Let it go.

Finally, you will always be divinely supported from an abundance point of view. You will receive the abundance exactly when you need it. It will come to you, and you never have to force anything. Trust in that and allow the universe to work on your behalf so you can be divinely supported in every moment and in perfect timing.

PART 3

Dealing with Outcomes

CHAPTER 9

Circumstances Versus State of Being

⟢

*For Your Reflection in the Mirror to Smile,
You Must Smile First*

— Bashar

If there is one quote by Bashar that you can keep repeating to yourself every single day, let it be this:

"Circumstances don't matter. Only state of being matters."

Repeat this and keep reminding yourself of this any time you manifest a circumstance that is not to your preference. Nothing happens to you. You are the painter of your picture. You are the star actor, writer, director and producer of your movie. No one else is.

If a circumstance you don't prefer is showing up, you have unknowingly created that. Don't go into victim mode. Don't blame the other person involved. Don't become negative and react. Look within and find the belief that has created that circumstance. Everything can be changed by changing yourself first.

As Bashar puts it, for your reflection in the mirror to smile back at you, you must smile first. How else can the reflection in the mirror change?

Follow your joy and use that as an opportunity to raise your vibration while your higher mind leads you to your desires. But, first, your higher mind may reveal to you what beliefs you may have that may be blocking the manifestation. So some unwanted manifestations may occur. It's a good thing! You know that you're on the right track because by clearing that roadblock, which can be done very easily, as we'll cover in Chapter 10, you can continue on your path and achieve all your desires.

It's an absolute win-win. You are happy as you follow your joy AND you're on your journey to all your desires. There's no waiting involved. You're living in every moment. The whole "follow your joy" formula is already part of your magnificent manifestations.

> I had an experience recently that was a circumstance I did not prefer. That's actually putting it lightly. It was an experience that I outright hated. I manifested a breakup. As I was writing these words, I kept getting the image of a donkey kicking me in the face. When I looked up the spiritual meaning of a donkey, one of the meanings was humility.

I laughed at the meaning because that perfectly describes what this experience was teaching me. Humility. Stay humble in the "not knowing" what deep-held beliefs we may be holding on to. I have been a conscious manifester for 17 years! We may think we get it all. But we don't always. I was sure that I had identified all my limiting subconscious beliefs around my relationship. Yet, as I was following my joy and was in the most positive of spaces, out of the blue, I manifested that breakup. At first, I went into victim mode (yes, after 17 years of doing this!) but then I went back and reminded myself that I am the full creator of my experience.

When I remembered that, I went back into a positive state. I realized that I was still holding on to certain beliefs and fears, resulting from past experiences where I was blindsided. Because of that fear, I unknowingly found myself focusing on the unwanted. It was the fear enforcing itself. I kept dismissing the fear, not knowing where it was coming from. If I had addressed that fear by questioning where it was coming from, I would have been able to release the subconscious belief that I would be blindsided.

But I didn't. And that's exactly what happened. That's why I needed that "negative" outcome to occur, so I could release that huge roadblock that was creating strain in my relationship.

Your desires WANT to manifest in exactly the way you imagine them and prefer them. YOU are keeping them away.

Humility is key. In some situations, we might be great manifesters, while in others, we unconsciously fall into our old victim mentality.

The idea is to never be hard on ourselves. Stay in a positive place no matter what. Certainly, this was also a reminder to me and a much-needed example for my book so we can all be reminded to release our ego, which thinks it knows everything.

The good news is that these circumstances are never permanent. Everything is fluid and can be changed. Sometimes instantly. You can never do permanent damage. Ever. Because of the concept of parallel realities. You have the power to shift in every single moment and focus on your preferred reality. This not only changes your future, but it changes your past as well. Your past only resides in your memory.

Any time the memory of what happened pops up and you feel compelled to blame the other person, go back and remind yourself that you painted the picture. They are just posing in your portrait. They did not paint themselves.

The people in your reality are your supporting actors and extras. They are waiting for all the cues from YOU. If you make the past irrelevant to you, it certainly will be irrelevant to them because the mirror always reflects back to you your state of being. Just get back up and keep moving forward because you just cleared a major roadblock to the extraordinary life you desire to live.

In my story, I can blame the other person for the breakup or I can get back on my feet and remind myself that I fully manifested it, and then determine what I would like to manifest with that person from this point forward.

Circumstances DO Matter

Although Bashar's quote states "circumstances don't matter," it does not mean that we should ignore these circumstances or deny that they exist. They DO matter in the sense that they are showing us that we have some inner beliefs that need to come to light. Do the work of digging in and bringing these to your conscious awareness. Do not ignore the circumstance, hoping it will go away by itself.

For example, let's say a married woman, through the experiences of her other married friends, begins to create a belief within her that "all men at some point cheat in their marriages." While she might not be conscious of it, the recurring experiences of her friends and her emotions around those situations have imprinted that belief in her subconscious.

As a result, she manifests just that in her own relationship. She can go into victim mode, blame him, and end the marriage, only to recreate the same experience with another person (as the person is gone but the belief isn't). Or she can dig into her subconscious and find out what inner beliefs have created that situation. By doing that, she can clear the belief and enforce more positive beliefs around her own relationship experiences, whether she chooses to stay or leave.

Whichever path she chooses, and only if she allows this experience to impact her, her hang-up right now may be that negative circumstance, which is stored as an experience in her memory, and she may be compelled to go back to that memory for self-victimization and a justification to blame others. Any time that happens, she needs to go back and remind herself that she created it. Period.

Do you fire the supporting actor in the movie for playing out the script exactly as you "unknowingly" wrote it? There is no one else conspiring or doing anything to us. We are conspiring and doing these things to ourselves. It may not be easy at first but, with practice, those circumstances become truly irrelevant.

Other Reasons for Non-preferred Circumstances

Underlying limiting beliefs are the most common reason why your unwanted circumstances manifest. But they are not the only reason.

Time-Lag Echoes

As you stabilize your state of being and your overall practiced vibration increases, you may, at times, manifest some "echoes" of your previous vibration.

As mentioned in a previous chapter, manifestations are instant in the spiritual realm. In the physical world, there is a time lag between intention and manifestation. Therefore, there might be a delay between the time you set the intention and/or change your state of being and the time the outer reality changes. It is crucial that during this period, you allow the manifestation to come to fruition without getting out of your positive state.

You can consider it as somewhat of a test on whether or not you have actually changed. If you do not react negatively to external circumstances, then you have changed. Remember, the reflection in the mirror cannot change unless you have changed first. If you have truly changed, then you will not react negatively to any negative outcomes that could potentially be echoes of a previously practiced vibration.

For example, you may have a terrible boss, whom you cannot tolerate. As you're reading this book, you think about your boss and come to realize that you have subconscious beliefs that "all bosses are horrible." The experiences over the past year with this boss have reinforced that belief. So it's a vicious cycle! But you decide to release that belief. Sure, it might be easier to move to a new job and start with a blank slate with a new boss, with whom you have no history. But how about you manifest it with your current boss? Now that you know that your inner beliefs attracted that behavior from your boss, you can shift your focus to all the times when your boss showed compassion or was nice (even if just momentarily).

Due to the time lag, you may not see the change in your boss' behavior right away. In fact, he may still be downright mean. By knowing that this is an echo of your previous state of being and beliefs, you can remain positive and not react. If you do that, it is guaranteed that you will start to see evidence of the changed behavior.

Contrast for Greater Clarity

Some negative outcomes are manifested for the purpose of contrast, which means getting clearer on what we want versus what we don't want. We spoke earlier about polarity, which is necessary for understanding ourselves and expanding our awareness and consciousness on what we prefer versus what we do not prefer. If it weren't for the dark, we would not understand the light. It is a natural part of the expansion of awareness.

As we go through life, we will experience circumstances that we do not prefer in order to get greater clarity on our desires and what we do prefer. It is part of the experience of "launching a new rocket of desire," as stated by Abraham-Hicks. It's a new opportunity to demonstrate your ability to create more of what you want and less of what you don't want.

As your vibration increases, your awareness also grows of the choice available to immediately shift towards what you do prefer (rather than maintaining focus on what you do not want or prefer).

It is never about "ignoring" what you don't prefer or pretending it's not there. In fact, as your vibration rises, your awareness of that negativity increases. But it's always about focusing your attention towards what you do want.

Often, if you are "on the fence" or undecided about your preferences, you wobble in your manifestations. Therefore, a negative manifestation would allow you to decide what you prefer so you no longer wobble. And you have the choice to immediately shift in that regard.

Finally, when it comes to what's happening in the world, you're not supposed to be in denial. You're supposed to observe the situation and focus on the opposite of it. It's never about looking at a negative situation through rose-colored glasses, which is what many people consider to be "positive thinking." In fact, those who have a positive practiced vibration are the ones that feel the negativity more than others. The key is to shift the focus from war to peace. By observing war, you don't deny that it's there, but you use that contrast to shift your focus towards peace (leaving out the "how" that can happen). When you do this, you help shift to a more peaceful earth, which itself is also shifting.

Focus on what you prefer to experience so that your external reality molds into a more preferred experience.

Highest Possible Version of a Manifestation

Often, when we set intentions, we rely on an image created by the physical mind of what that manifestation should look like. Our higher mind then works to guide us so we realign our vibration and manifest the highest possible version of our desire that is guaranteed to fulfill us. The physical mind cannot conceive this but the higher mind can. Therefore, it is important to not remain attached to the physical image we've created of what our manifestation should look like and how it should come about.

In order to have a better and higher appreciation for our ultimate manifestation, we may manifest certain people, opportunities, situations, and experiences that will allow us to become fuller versions of ourselves so that we may ultimately become more vibrationally compatible with our desire.

For example, if you want to attract a new relationship but your practiced vibration is not yet in an ideal state, by following the formula of Chapter 7, your higher mind will guide you through a path of general experiences that may help you raise your vibration first in order to manifest a "better version" of your ideal relationship. Otherwise, you may attract a relationship that is less than ideal based on your practiced vibration. This is all part of the manifestation and there is no "delay." You are just attracting your ideal relationship in its highest form.

Alternatively, your practiced vibration might be high but you have certain hidden beliefs about self-worth that would impact your manifestation or cause you to manifest a relationship where you are not loved in the way you would like to be. Again, by following your joy, you allow your higher mind to guide you in a way that brings these beliefs of self-worth to your awareness so you can clear them. This may happen by being guided to do some meditation or attend a self-love retreat or simply attracting a less than ideal relationship that can then shed light on your inner beliefs. Everything you experience is part of the manifestation. Use these circumstances to build more self-awareness so you experience your manifestations in their highest form.

Don't Sweat the Small Stuff

If we monitor how frequently we tend to react to the small stuff, we'll be surprised how much we often jeopardize our own state of being over the small things. The book *Don't Sweat the Small Stuff...* by Richard Carlson is a wonderful book that really helped me notice and shift those reactions within myself. These small outbursts or mood shifts really impact our overall chronic vibration. The less reactive we are in general, the more we allow our vibration to stabilize. And as our vibration stabilizes, we are either less bothered or we don't manifest these circumstances altogether.

In the past, I used to be quite reactive to everyday circumstances. I had set an intention to practice being more present and less reactive, especially since I understood how much more valuable it was to remain in a "feeling good" space regardless of whether someone was right or not.

Of course, I had to prove that I had changed!

One time, shortly after I had set the intention to become less reactive, I manifested an experience with a social media provider. Although I was having a very cordial interaction with him, he was being rude in his approach. I did not like it, but I remained very centered and present. I did not have the urge to react as I normally would have, although

I did feel the discomfort of it, especially since I was paying him (my belief was that, as a paying client, I should get great service). I knew this was my opportunity to show that I had changed. There was progress there because, even though I did feel bothered on the inside, I did not react.

The next time, I manifested mostly kind behavior in the face of some random unpleasant comments, although they were less rude than those that had been said to me the first time. This time, I not only did not react, but I also did not feel anything. It was very empowering, and I still asserted myself lovingly without taking myself out of alignment.

After that time, the interaction changed 180 degrees, and I started to only manifest great experiences and service from him.

It's a given that we cannot always control our reactions. Sometimes, we just have bad days and it's okay. The key is what we're doing most of the time and learning to gently shift ourselves back into alignment. Remember to always be kind to yourself and allow yourself to be human.

⊷⊷● ●⊶⊶

In conclusion, circumstances that you manifest are not what matter. It's how you react to them that does.

No matter what manifests, remain in a positive space in order to discern the purpose of that circumstance. It might just be a time-lag echo; at other times, it is an indication of a hidden belief that needs to be released.

Circumstances are not permanent and can always be changed. Do not get discouraged by what appears as "something wrong" or a "lack of progress." You are always on the right path if you make your practiced vibration your top priority, for every step of the way is a key component of your ideal manifestation.

When you learn to do that, you will truly have mastered the manifestation process and can allow the wave of resulting synchronicities to take you through a truly fulfilling life experience.

CHAPTER 10

Your Reflection

The Power of the Subconscious

-»‖⦿ ⦿‖«-

"All that we are is the result of what we have thought.
The mind is everything. What we think, we become."

— The Buddha

I used to think that by believing that "everything is possible," we can attract anything we set our mind to. However, one positive thought or belief alone may not be powerful enough to supersede other limiting and possibly contradictory subconscious beliefs that we surely have and are not aware of.

It's important to understand that both your subconscious and unconscious minds are not below your conscious mind, as the terms may indicate and give the conscious mind the idea that it is "in charge." They are above the conscious mind in terms of vibrational frequency. The unconscious mind, which operates at the highest frequency, is above the subconscious mind, which is, in turn, higher than the conscious mind.

The unconscious mind contains the most repressed thoughts, memories and beliefs, while the subconscious mind is the stage between the conscious and unconscious mind.

Whatever thoughts and beliefs are present at unconscious and subconscious levels are very powerful and will always supersede our conscious thoughts and beliefs. Our subconscious minds always reflect back what's imprinted within them without any discernment of whether these notions make sense or not – our subconscious minds just take the orders.

By following the formula of Chapter 7, these subconscious beliefs and definitions may start to come to light through unwanted manifestations in order to reveal to us that we are holding on to some limiting beliefs.

Merely becoming aware of these beliefs is enough to release them so we no longer attract the unwanted manifestations. The experiences you've had reflect that belief and reinforce it. But it was always the belief that came first. Although we will be covering how beliefs are often born, you do not have to dig into why you have that belief because it doesn't really matter.

Once you do that, you will no longer manifest the circumstances created by that belief.

But let's first understand what beliefs are.

Definition of Beliefs

Some definitions of beliefs in the dictionary are as follows:
- "an acceptance that something exists or is true; a firmly held opinion." – *Oxford Dictionary*
- "something that is accepted, considered to be true, or held as an opinion; something believed." – *Merriam-Webster*

None of the definitions state a belief as "fact." But we may believe something to be "fact" because we keep experiencing the reflection of it in our experience. The important point to understand is that your reality is a consequence of your inner beliefs and not vice versa. The belief always came first.

How Beliefs Are Born

As we go through life, we accumulate thousands of beliefs about all aspects of life. Many of these beliefs start early in childhood, when we are highly impressionable, as we adopt the beliefs of influential people in our circle, such as our parents, teachers, friends and other family members.

As we adopt the beliefs of other people, we start to experience manifestations that reflect those beliefs, thereby reinforcing them as true.

Life Themes

At a soul level, before coming into the physical experience, we agreed to explore certain life themes. These themes will reflect the areas where we may experience more struggle. You will generally know what themes you have chosen to explore because they are in an area that has repeating patterns or is more difficult to let go of.

This will generally play a role in the early belief systems that we adopt and become harder to let go of as we experience life.

Types of Beliefs
Positive Versus Negative Beliefs

To keep matters simple, in this book, a negative belief can be defined as a practiced thought that acts as a barrier to our own expansion. Limiting thoughts are what prevent us from becoming more authentically ourselves.

However, not all beliefs are negative. There are some beliefs that are positive and serve us! These are the ones we should reinforce. For example, believing that the "universe is abundant" is a positive belief that benefits us.

The key is to invest in positive beliefs and to uncover (and, consequently, release) our negative beliefs. The latter is not always easy because when it comes to negative beliefs, they will often reinforce themselves in a way that makes it seem like no other belief is possible. They will use tricks to create fear within us so we cannot choose a positive belief.

Once you become aware of the tricks of negative belief systems, you will be better equipped to handle the fear that comes up and understand that you are actually on the verge of releasing those negative beliefs.

Our beliefs can be divided into three main categories:
- Beliefs about self.
- Beliefs about others.
- Beliefs about life and circumstances.

Beliefs About Self

The most common limiting beliefs are about us. People often find it uncomfortable to dig deep into their belief systems about themselves because they are afraid that they might be true.

Common beliefs about self include:
- I'm unworthy.
- I'm incompetent.
- I'm not good enough.
- I'm not smart enough.
- I can't do it.
- I don't know how to do it.
- I'm too fat/thin.
- I'm too tall/short.
- I don't deserve it.
- I have nothing to offer.
- And the list goes on and on...

In her book *You Can Heal Your Life*, Louise Hay stated that the most common limiting belief people hold is "I'm not good enough." It's really a catch-all for every negative belief one can have about themselves. And many times, it's about pure self-love.

People experience self-love issues because they believe the voice of the ego, which is very commonly self-critical and compares itself to others. They end up associating with that voice and holding those definitions as true. They consequently manifest experiences that reflect those beliefs and reinforce them further.

Yet, by disidentifying from the ego mind and becoming aware of that infinite creator within us (our inner being or higher mind) that is separate from the thinking mind, we can realize that the negative words and thoughts are just illusions, and any limiting idea we have about ourselves can be changed instantly. And when we do that, the reality starts to shift to reinforce our new preferable identity.

So, here are some examples of how these self-beliefs may manifest:

Self-Belief	Examples of How It Manifests
I'm unworthy.	You manifest jobs where you are underpaid or paid less than others. You manifest relationships with partners who don't treat you well. You manifest friends who don't value your time or opinion (they're always late, or don't take your opinion into consideration when making plans).

Self-Belief	Examples of How It Manifests
I'm not smart enough.	You manifest situations where you don't appear smart to others. You manifest situations where you can't do something or you don't have the required skill to do the job right. You manifest situations where people tell you you're not smart.
I'm too fat/thin.	You manifest someone who doesn't like your weight or doesn't want to be with you because of your weight. You attract relationships or people who criticize your weight ("You've gained weight," "You're too thin!"). You manifest even more weight gain/loss.

Remember, those are just your OPINIONS about yourself and opinions are not facts. You consider them facts because you attract the situations that reflect them and reinforce them. *It always starts with the belief.*

You are never a victim. Ever. Everyone is YOU projected out-wards. You experience the behaviors from others that are reflec-tive of your inner beliefs. You are the star, writer, director and producer of your own movie. Everyone you interact with is just a supporting actor or "extras" in your movie, taking cues from you and only you!

They are doing the same in THEIR own parallel reality, where a ver-sion of you is present and playing the role of a supporting actor in their movie.

Once you really get this, your life will change forever because you start to realize the extent of your inner power.

Change your inner beliefs and your outer reality has to shift.

Beliefs About Others

When it comes to how other people show up in your reality, as you get to know certain people, you start to develop opinions about them based on their actions and behaviors, which are (ironically!) the result of general beliefs and preconceived ideas you may have about yourself or people in general. As they continue to mirror back to you non-preferred actions and behaviors, you begin to define them based on who you perceive them to be.

This then becomes further reinforced as they must continue to mirror back to you all the attitudes, qualities, actions and behaviors that you do not prefer. It really becomes a vicious cycle.

The core belief is always about YOU. Other people are always reflecting back to you a belief that you have about yourself or preconceived limiting beliefs you have about people in general.

When it comes to preconceived limiting beliefs, these often come from generalizations about groups of people. For example:
- All/most bosses are mean.
- All/most people from X nationality are rude.
- People from this country do x.
- Most good men are taken.
- Most women are looking for a rich husband.
- Etc.

As a result, you attract just that, even if you've just met that person. They will show up based on your generalizations and definitions because your physical reality and everyone in it are all just a reflection of your subconscious beliefs.

Beliefs About Circumstances

People also make negative conclusions about circumstances in general. For example:
- Finding a job is difficult during a recession.
- Money doesn't grow on trees.
- There is never enough.
- Money is the root of all evil.

Again, this always reflects back in your reality. That is why it is important to not always engage in these negative conversations with others because you never want to be influenced by other people's limiting beliefs about what's possible.

Looking at your physical reality, you can conclude which life areas are impacted by negative beliefs. For example, if you are barely making ends meet, then there must be some limiting beliefs around money.

Sometimes it's a combination of beliefs about self, others and circumstances.

Regardless of the type of belief, a good question to ask yourself is this:

What would I have to believe about myself, others or circumstances in order to be manifesting this situation?

However, you cannot assume that a given manifestation will have the same underlying belief for everyone. These will always be different for different people because much of our beliefs come from our upbringing as well as our values and personal experiences, which are unique to us.

> One example is a client who was having difficulty in her love life and that was impacting her ability to express her passions. She was investing a great deal of time, energy and focus on her love for a man, who was not available.
>
> At face value, one would expect that her limiting beliefs would include any of the following:
> • All good men are taken.

- I am not good enough (therefore, I deserve only "part of someone").
- I don't deserve to be number one.
- I don't deserve to be chosen.

However, when we dug deep, we discovered, surprisingly, that none of these were her core beliefs. As we persisted in uncovering the root cause of her manifestation, it came down to one major belief she had and that was "normal relationships are boring."

It was a huge a-ha for her and, in fact, that belief also caused most of her relationships to be short-lived, ending when the initial passion phased out. When she understood why her physical reality was manifesting in that way, she was able to release the negative belief, and she also worked on enforcing more positive beliefs about relationships.

"I do not fix problems. I fix my thinking. Then problems fix themselves."

— Louise Hay

Of course, it helps to be proactive and run an exhaustive list of all limiting beliefs that you may have. But you won't feel compelled to do it when it doesn't seem relevant in the moment. You might disregard certain beliefs as not having any impact, until you actually manifest a situation that reveals you hold them true.

Sometimes you will receive cues about hidden beliefs through your dreams, which are also manifestations. This doesn't require diving too deep for interpretation. It's often an obvious situation that you don't prefer, such as dreaming about a job loss or breakup. This can be a cue that you have some beliefs around that situation that must be released and it's best to dig into this before you manifest the situation in your physical reality.

With regards to my own breakup, I actually dreamt about it two months earlier, but rather than digging into the underlying beliefs I may have had, I focused on remaining in a positive space. Humility is key. Don't assume that you have nailed and released all your inner beliefs. If you're dreaming it, there's something there. That is a perfect example of a situation where I could have dug deep to avoid the real-life manifestation.

Belief Systems

Oftentimes, different beliefs work together to reinforce one another, creating belief systems around a certain life area. Typically, there will be one core or fundamental belief and multiple secondary beliefs tied to that core belief.

If you let go of a secondary belief, which exists only to support the fundamental belief, you may continue to attract the undesired circumstances because you have not identified the root belief that was the basis for that secondary belief.

You may not know which is the core belief and which is the secondary belief but you must keep digging until you find it.

Example

A woman is always strained for money and can't seem to get out of that situation. When digging deep, she uncovers that she has the following beliefs:

- I don't need a lot of money to be happy.
- Money is not important.
- It's selfish to want money.
- Money is not a priority.

Despite letting these beliefs go, she keeps manifesting financial lack, indicating that she is still holding on to a core belief around money. After some further reflection, she discovers that she has a belief that "Money is the root of all evil." When she realizes that, she understands that this core belief is the basis for all the additional beliefs she has around money. Since she believed that it was the root of all evil, she built a number of supporting beliefs around money to further reinforce that core belief.

In order for her to change her relationship with money, and attract abundance, she must find the core belief and release that. In this case:

"Money is the root of all evil."

By bringing this into her conscious awareness, she can automatically release it because she can see that it is far from true.

Working with Beliefs

When it comes to working with beliefs, we always want to release negative beliefs and reinforce positive ones.

Releasing Negative Beliefs

In order to release a negative belief, it only takes bringing these beliefs to your conscious awareness in order to let them go. You go beyond the belief just by knowing it's there, and understanding that these are just illusionary thoughts and opinions we have chosen to hold as true.

Reinforcing Positive Beliefs

When it comes to reinforcing positive beliefs, the key is to imprint these new beliefs into our subconscious mind to create a healthier and more empowering self-image.

This has played a big role in my own life, allowing me to build a positive self-concept and attract the experiences that reflect that.

Reinforcing positive beliefs can be done in one of the following ways:

1. Repetition.
    Have you ever driven yourself to work and wondered how you actually got there? Back when I lived in Beirut, I was driving my family to my aunt's house, which involved taking almost the same route as my usual drive to work, except my work location required a right turn at the end of the route while my aunt's home was on

a left turn. As I was driving, I was focused on the radio and was suddenly interrupted by my dad, who jokingly asked, "Are you driving us to work?" Without realizing it, my subconscious mind drove us to work.

Repetition of anything – actions, verbal words, thoughts – will imprint it into our subconscious mind. This is how habits are formed. It is said that through 21 days, a repeated action, word or thought becomes a habit.

Knowing this, you can use the power of repetition to imprint positive statements (affirmations) into your subconscious mind so that they become beliefs. This can be done either consciously (by repeating statements verbally, in writing or in your thoughts), or subconsciously.

Some examples of positive statements that can be repeated and imprinted as beliefs into the subconscious mind are the following:

- I excel in all that I do.
- I love myself and I am loved for who I am.
- I am always supported in the pursuit of my dreams and passions.
- I excel at doing work I love.
- Success comes very naturally to me as I pursue my passions.
- Abundance flows to me with great ease.
- I always have enough money.
- I am well-organized and I manage my time efficiently.
- I am beautiful, inside out.
- I am lean, fit and healthy.
- My metabolism is high and I burn fat easily.

- I am healthy, and I look great.
- I radiate love and love comes back to me.
- The more I love myself, the more others love me. I am worthy of love.
- I attract partners that resonate with me.

Conscious Repetition

When repeating the statements consciously, it is important that you feel good while saying them. Feel the power of these positive statements and consider them done. If saying them causes you to cringe and remember that it's not currently evidenced in your reality, then they will be counterproductive, and it may be better to opt for the subconscious option.

Subconscious Repetition

Did you know that every day, information is being fed into your subconscious mind without your conscious awareness? Everything you see with your eyes or hear with your ears is being captured by your subconscious mind whether you are conscious of it or not. That is the very basis of advertising!

This same process can be used to repeat positive thoughts directly into your subconscious mind so that, with time, they become beliefs. The reason I love this method is because it takes the conscious mind out of the equation. So when words are repeated at a subliminal level into your subconscious mind, the conscious mind cannot interrupt and say, "Hey, that's not true."

That is why it seems almost "miraculous" when the very words you are subconsciously repeating manifest. In this way, your subconscious and unconscious minds are much more powerful than your conscious mind. By simply surpassing our conscious thoughts and not activating them, we can create new belief systems that best serve us.

The most common subliminal messages come in the form of meditation audios, which lower your brainwave activity for better access to your subconscious mind and then feed the positive messages into your subconscious.

Check out my website for more information on subliminal messages.

2. Experiences Reinforced with Emotions.
   As mentioned in an earlier chapter, the subconscious mind does not know the difference between what is real and what isn't real as it has no access to our physical reality experience. It only knows what is fed to it.

   Therefore, whether you are having a real-life experience or visualizing or reflecting through memories, the subconscious mind does not know the difference. Experiences are just neutral situations we have in life. What makes them powerful is the emotion that is attached to them.

   That is why we will always remember the happiest and unhappiest moments in our lives, as the emotion gives the experience a magnetic charge, causing it to be imprinted into our subconscious minds. Therefore, these experiences – and the meaning we give to them – become very powerful inner drivers.

Using the techniques shared in this book to imprint intentions would be exactly how you imprint positive experiences into your subconscious mind.

The beauty of all this is that as you change your inner beliefs, you start to attract the experiences in your physical reality, which further reinforce these beliefs, especially when you experience them with joy, love and a sense of fulfillment. That is why it is incredibly important to maintain a positive state of being, no matter the outcome, so that your negative emotions (caused by your negative reaction) will not imprint those experiences in a negative way into your subconscious mind.

⊸═◉ ◉═⊷

As a conclusion for this chapter and book, here is a quick recap of the most important points to consider:

- You are a spiritual being having a physical experience.
- You came here to experience the creation process and to express your uniqueness, which is a new and essential perspective required for the "whole" to be complete.
- Your true life purpose is to express your unique qualities and manifest your desires as fully as you can so that you live a life that is extraordinary, ecstatic, expansive, joyful, curious, imaginative and loving.
- Your physical reality is always a reflection of your subconscious mind. Everything and everyone is YOU projected outwards.
- In every moment, you have the opportunity to shift to a new and more preferred parallel reality.

- You are always being guided by your higher mind through the physical sensation of excitement, passion and love.
- In this movie you call "life," you are the lead actor, writer, producer and director. The only free will that matters and is relevant in your movie is your own free will.

In closing, I would like for you to consider the following question and to set an intention in writing on how you would like your life to be different.

If you were to fast-forward in your mind to six months from now, and you imagine that you have implemented all the teachings of this book, how would your life be different?

(Let your imagination flow, for you are the writer, lead actor, producer, and director of your own unique life movie).

_____

_____

_____

_____

_____

_____

_____

Becoming You

_____

_____

_____

_____

_____

_____

_____

_____

_____

_____

_____

_____

_____

_____

_____

_____

_____

_____

_____

_____

_____

_____

_____

_____

_____

_____

_____

_____

Becoming You

_____

_____

_____

_____

_____

_____

_____

_____

_____

_____

_____

_____

_____

_____

Acknowledgments

This acknowledgment page is for all the people who have helped me become more ME and played an important role in me putting these words in writing.

To my family:
- Mom and Dad for your unconditional love and always supporting my passions and decisions, even when they didn't always make sense!
- My sister, Reem, for supporting me unconditionally and using your magical healing skills to bring me back into balance.
- My brother, Ahmad, and sister-in-law, Lamees, for always encouraging me and supporting my decisions.
- My nieces, Aya and Hana, for all the love and joy that you bring into my life.

To my coaches:
- Moustafa Hamwi for pushing me to get this book done!
- Regan Hillyer for showing me what's possible and helping me get my new message out.
- Gabby Bernstein for guiding me in putting words on paper and telling my story.

To my friends:

- Reeman, Alison and Francesca for infusing me with positivity whenever I needed it and being my biggest cheerleaders.
- Nuhad and Raya for always believing in me and cheering me on.
- Erica for giving me the idea to write a book!

To all my soulmates:

- For unknowingly triggering me and inspiring me to become the best version of myself.

Author Bio

Mona Shibel is a Consultant and Manifestation and Soul Realignment Coach with seventeen years of experience in conscious manifesting.

When she first learned about the Law of Attraction in 2006, she realized that she had already been unknowingly manifesting intentions in her own life, including creating a major shift in 2005 when she moved from Beirut to Dubai.

Mona started her career in the field of banking in 1995 and shifted into consulting in 2005. She started her own entrepreneurial journey in 2008 when she established an online business, which was fully the outcome of her conscious manifesting. As a result, Mona was able to achieve success for her business, growing it into a regional bilingual website with high monthly traffic and attracting an equity investor for her business. She also quit her full-time job, grew her consulting career as a sought-after independent consultant, and created a freedom-based life working on her own terms. She also started a coaching business in 2013 that offered business coaching services and has since shifted fully into spiritual-based coaching focused on manifesting and soul realignment.

Through her own experiences, and personal growth, she has peeled back the layers on who she really is and how she can joyfully and authentically express herself at every step.

Mona is currently based in Dubai, living her dreams and following her own joy in every decision along the way. Through her coaching, Mona helps clients become the highest versions of themselves so they can create and live the extraordinary lives that are their birthrights.

CPSIA information can be obtained
at www.ICGtesting.com
Printed in the USA
BVHW072202030222
627978BV00001B/45

9 781761 240006